Freedom
Through Health

REVISED AND UPDATED

Terry Shepherd Friedmann, M.D.

Manufactured in the United States of America.
This edition published by Harvest Publishing,
P.O. Box 33270, Northglenn, CO 80233-3270

10 9 8 7 6 5 4 3 2 1

Edited by Karla Olson, Via Press
Cover and interior design by
Gopa Design and Illustration

ISBN 0-9638366-8-4
Library of Congress Catalog Card Number: 98-70221

The medical information and procedures contained in
this book are not intended as an substitute for consulting with your physician. Any attempt to diagnose or
treat an illness should come under the direction of a
physician who is familiar with and trained in medicine,
procedures, and treatment, preferably with a knowledge
of holistic medicine.

This book is a reference work based upon research by
the author. The opinions expressed herein are those of
the author and are not necessarily those of the publisher.

DEDICATION

This book is dedicated to my wife, Jean-Marie, who provided the encouragement and environment that enabled me to write this book. I also dedicate it to my patients, who were my best teachers when it came to the knowledge and cases needed to make this an informative and interesting book.

Terry Shepherd Friedmann, M.D.

Contents

PREFACE

Why Did I Revise this Book?

WHEN I PUBLISHED *Freedom Through Health* in 1993, it represented the latest concepts of holistic medicine. Five years later, however, much research has been done and many new facts have been discovered that promote healing. The amount of medical information in alternative fields doubles every three-and-a-half years. Therefore, in order to encompass all of the new knowledge to better improve health and save lives, I felt it was important as well as timely to share this new information.

In addition, I have extensively studied the application of pure essential oils and the science of aromatherapy in healing the body, mind, and spirit. Since aromatherapy is relatively new to the United States, in 1996 I traveled to Turkey and the University of Ege in Izmir. Here, as in France and England, the knowledge of the science of healing with essential oils is advanced. I have applied these healing techniques in my clinic, with significant positive clinical results.

Another rapidly growing medical speciality is anti-aging. There has been tremendous progress in medicine that has enabled physicians to reverse the aging process through the use of newly discovered nutrients as well as the use of specific hormones, whose actions we now better understand. There are a growing number of people among us who accept that their potential for longevity is presently at their finger tips. Not only that, but people expect to live a full and active life. I have consequently written a chapter discussing this topic.

Lastly, there is a significant challenge to us that is the result of new virulent diseases occurring throughout our planet. Furthermore, an increasing number of persons are experiencing immune system dysfunction. Therefore, their bodies' defenses against these debilitating and sometimes fatal diseases is greatly impaired. One of the areas I have stressed in my practice is methods of strengthening the immune system. Best of all, I have created this by utilizing natural remedies. I have included a completely revised chapter addressing the immune system and explaining how to maximize its function.

In summary, the revised book has been streamlined and updated and is a wonderful source of information that one can utilize to achieve optimal health and longevity.

FOREWORD

by Garry F. Gordon,
M.D., D.O., M.D.(H.)

I HAVE WORKED with Dr. Friedmann for many years, and have the highest regard for his dedication to improving the health of his fellow man. The practical advice contained in this book can benefit almost everyone today, because we all are operating far below our maximum potential. We are all very busy, and still tend to rely on medical relief of symptoms rather than locating the causes of our health problems.

It gives me great pleasure to have this opportunity to endorse the highly practical and cost effective concepts so well explained in *Freedom Through Health*. Dr. Friedmann's expertise with essential oils opens a new era of cost effective home health care, as he puts them into a more comprehensive integrative approach to achieving optimal health.

As the president of the International College of Advanced Longevity Medicine (ICALM) I was particularly pleased to see the practical suggestions on reversing the aging process contained in this book. There is much that can be done in anti-aging/longevity medicine, and Dr. Friedmann provides a good, basic foundation for the exciting developments in controlling human aging that will soon become widely available to everyone.

— Dr. Garry F. Gordon

FOREWORD

by Gladys Taylor McGarey, M.D., M.D.(H)

Past president of the Arizona Board of Homeopathic Medical Examiners
Co-founder and Director of the Scottsdale Holistic Medical Group
Past president of the American Holistic Medical Association

IT WAS DURING THE WEE HOURS of the morning almost twenty years ago that two of my colleagues and I were waiting for one of my patients to have her baby and were in a discussion in the doctor's room. The conversation was revolving around the condition of medicine at that time. One of my colleagues said, "The problem is that all the fun has gone out of medicine," and my other colleague responded with, "You're so right. There's no way that I would encourage my daughter to go into medicine."

During the intervening twenty years, I thought a lot about these two comments and realized that at the present time the situation has not improved but has really become more of a problem, not only for physicians but for patients. Medicine, which was a noble profession when I first began practicing in 1946, has become a difficult, often unrewarding job. Those of us who went into medicine because we wanted to serve, find our hands tied, so it's very difficult to do for our patients what we feel is best for them and we find ourselves practicing defensive medicine.

In spite of all of the above, I still find that there is "fun in medicine." I think the reason has to do with a deep knowing that when I do my job the best way I know how, the patient does the healing within their very being. This Dr. Friedmann has addressed beautifully in this book. We find ourselves working with a patient who happens to have a disease process and no matter how difficult that process is to diagnose, how impossible the disease to treat, we still have a patient who is a living human being who has responses and emotions and life force which is always, even until the last breath, a dynamic, exciting force.

In the field of medicine today there are many ancient therapeutic modalities that are becoming available to us. Among them are acupuncture, homeopathy, and nutritional concept and massage. Also available is aromatherapy, in which the use of essential oils works at a deep cellular but also vibratory level. Dr. Friedmann has developed and is presenting to us ways in which we can use these oils. They help to balance body, mind, and spirit.

If all of us, physicians and patients alike, would use the program of Five Rs which is outlined in this book and supports and repairs our immune system, I truly believe that all of us would be healthier, happier, and better human beings. These principles are not difficult to follow and could be adapted in every household.

Dr. Terry Friedmann's book is a wonderful example of how the art of medicine can be practiced. It simply and clearly lays out ways where patients can take care of many things themselves and we as physicians can work with them in the healing process.

I am delighted to have this book to offer to my patients.

— Dr. Gladys Taylor McGarey

Section One

THE PHILOSOPHY OF HOLISTIC MEDICINE

CHAPTER 1

The Philosophy
of Holistic Medicine

THE COST OF GOOD HEALTH

BACK IN 1977 I heard the surgeon general, Dr. Julius Lippmann, proclaim that we must change the way medicine is practiced in the United States. At that time medical costs were approximately $300 billion dollars annually, and he was convinced that these costs would escalate significantly in the future unless action was taken immediately.

What did Dr. Lippmann recommend? That instead of spending only 6 percent of the annual health dollars on patient education and preventive medicine with 85 percent going to crisis medicine and 9 percent to chronic illness, the money should be redistributed. It would pay off quickly, he argued, if we as a country prioritized our resources. At least 15 percent of the expenditures should be devoted to education and preventive medicine with appropriately less to the other areas of health care.

I agree with Dr. Lippman that we need to see commitment in changing the basic way medicine is conceived. We must stop emphasizing crisis care—patching up the body when seriously advanced disease has occurred. We must intervene instead at both a preventive level and a deeper level.

However, this philosophy takes self responsibility. One must care enough about oneself to develop good habits that prevent serious diseases from occurring. This involves dealing with all levels of the person — emotional, mental, and physical, as well as spiritual. These all have great importance in the development of good health.

Also, instead of relying heavily on drugs and surgery, we should consider more natural approaches, such as a good diet and the use of vitamins and minerals and natural herbs. We should avoid those things in our environment that cause disease: chemical pollution, electromagnetic pollution, improper diet, and a sedentary lifestyle. We should learn to handle stress better. We need to take the time to be in contact with our inner self and our creator.

Believing that I could make a difference and therefore help my patients, I sought out these philosophies. I met with many like-minded physicians and in 1978 we formed the American Holistic Medical Association (AHMA). This is an organization that views people as totally integrated at all levels, including body, mind, and spirit.

🌿 Holistic Health

The AHMA considers holistic health to be a state of well-being in which an individual's body, mind, emotions, and spirit are in harmony with and guided by an awareness of society, nature, and the universe. According to the AHMA, holistic medicine is a system of medical care that emphasizes personal responsibility and fosters a cooperative relationship among all those involved, leading toward optimal attunement of body, mind, emotions, and spirit.

Holistic medicine encompasses all safe modalities of diagnosis and treatment, including the use of medication and surgery, and emphasizes the necessity of looking at the whole person, including analysis of physical, nutritional, environmental, emotional, spiritual, and life-style values. Holistic medicine particularly focuses upon patient education and responsibility in the healing process.

The AHMA promotes a philosophy that physicians in all areas of medicine can be holistically oriented. All physicians may benefit from a basic understanding of the principles of nutrition, exercise, and stress management and should have a continued awareness of the physical, emotional, mental, and spiritual nature of the whole person while practicing in a variety of specialties.

When the AHMA was established we believed that we could make an impact on the direction of medicine in the United States. Now, almost twenty years later, we are told by the government that the cost of health care in the United States could reach $1 trillion a year, many times the cost in 1977.

Most of all, health and longevity are not improving. People are using drugs and surgery more than ever, while very little money is being spent on education and preventive medicine.

There is now a serious problem posed by the Food and Drug Administration's (FDA's) attempts to over-regulate the individual's use of natural vitamins, minerals, and herbs. There are also significant efforts by insurance companies to exclude preventive health and education and the use of natural and inexpensive remedies, while they ignore the benefits of good nutrition. At the same time they are paying for huge medical claims due to hospitalizations, surgery, and pharmaceutical products.

This discrepancy came to my attention when I had occasion to meet with a insurance provider who refused to reimburse one of my patient's for medical services that I had provided. During the year prior to my treating her, the patient had suffered chronic medical ailments that had required her hospitalization numerous time. We explained that this patient's health was good now and that we were saving the insurance company money because she was better. They responded that they did not reimburse for natural medical procedures.

This puzzled me, at least until I discussed the case with Dr. Norman Shealy. He claimed in his book *Third Party* that during the last fifty years there has been an unwritten agreement between hospitals and insurance providers to reimburse the hospitals for most services performed in hospitals—to "scratch each other's back," so to speak.

It became obvious to me that in this agreement the insurance providers have a separate agenda.

If the insurance providers paid the hospitals for the patients' medical claims, then at the end of the year the insurance companies could go to the state insurance commissions with their track records and request a premium increase. A premium increase translates into more profit for the insurance carriers as well as the hospitals.

❧ But Is Our Health Better?

We as a country have dropped way below the rest of the industrially developed nations in infant mortality rate as well as other health problems. Acquired Immune Deficiency Syndrome (AIDS) is spreading rapidly and taking its toll on our citizenry. Because of our generally poor health habits our immune systems are overtaxed and dysfunctional.

Our government is complaining about the medical care crisis in this country. Unfortunately, an example of their answer to preventive medecine is a more extensive vaccination program throughout the country. That solves very few problems and may in fact create very serious ones.

There is a theory that many infectious diseases have cycles. The infection peaks among the population then declines and almost disappears, in a pattern similar to a bell curve. So whether we vaccinated or not, the disease would eventually disappear.

In addition, I and other physicians have found a connection between the time of vaccination and both hyperactivity and mental slowness. The statistics reveal that in some school districts 25 to 30 percent of the students are on Ritalin for hyperactivity. What is the reason for this? Could it be in fact due to the high rate of vaccination in this country? Could it also in fact be due to our childrens' excessive intake of refined sugar?

In my opinion a superior quality diet as well as increased use of natural products to improve the immune system is the preferred way to change our country's disease rates.

🌸 LIVE YOUR LIFE TO THE FULLEST

Yes, we are in the midst of a real crisis. However, I am convinced that it is not too late. We must all make a commitment to take responsibility for our lives. We must investigate for ourselves a safe and effective program in which we can achieve excellent health, one that shows there is hope!

I am convinced that we are on the verge of a new medicine—a new consciousness. We can all see a paradigm shift occurring in medicine. However, we must wake up and be willing to change our beliefs about how things must be done. Just because they were done "that way" in the past, doesn't make it a valid way to go today. Eventually all of us will require some degree of health or medical intervention during this lifetime.

The kind of doctor you choose is dependent upon your experience, knowledge, and personal needs. I hope that after you read this book you will choose a holistically trained physician. However, most important is that knowledge allows you to make the best decision you can about your health and life. Being in good health gives you freedom to live your life the way you feel it should be lived. Ultimately you should strive to be free of disease and live your life to the fullest.

🌸 ORGANIZATION OF THIS BOOK

I have chosen to break this book into three major sections. The first part is "The Philosophy of Holistic Medicine." To understand how holistic therapies work, it is essential that you understand the basic principles of health and healing and why disease happens. Without this concept it is difficult to get to the point where you have "freedom through health." For some, these concepts are all new, but, in fact, they are rooted in the principles of healing that have been known and practiced by our ancestors. These concepts have occurred in many cultures for thousands of years.

Once we understand the holistic philosophy we are ready to discuss the "Diseases of the 21st Century." This second section gives the formulas and tells how to approach some of the more common degenerative and infectious diseases and conditions.

In the third part, I pose the question "Where do we go from here?" What is some of the general information we should know in order to achieve self responsibility and, as a result, a higher, more balanced state of consciousness and health. Are we truly "our brother's keeper," as some biblical texts indicate? If so, then when we are well informed and functioning at the best level in our daily lives, we are better able to assist those around us, whomever they may be. Here I also discuss ways to reverse the aging process.

✿ SUMMARY OF PART I

What is the true cause of disease and illness? What are the factors that play a role in this process? Why do we get sick to begin with? Part I attempts to answer these questions and more. It defines the dimensions of the human being. It discusses being out of balance or harmony with our environment and how this leads to disease. Many of the more traditional therapies are discussed and how they have an impact on today's health.

Chapter 2

The Spirituality of Holism

My Quest

In 1975 I decided that my approach to medicine had to change. Even though I had a large, successful medical practice and was practicing "by the book," the results were not satisfying.

First, there was the wonderful little lady who kept getting one post-surgical complication after another until she was an invalid. I could not fully answer her family's questions concerning the causes of her escalating problems, and the answers I could give them were not reasonable. Medical school and post-graduate training simply had not prepared us doctors for some of these situations. Patients want simple answers and magic bullets and, naturally, expect physicians to supply them. Because of a lack of answers, I was motivated to begin a quest.

A New Organization

To satisfy my own curiosity, I traveled all over the country seeking information from other doctors, and I eventually found a group of physicians who felt as I did. As I noted earlier, we formed the American Holistic Medical Association in 1978. I served as a board member for 14 years.

❧ The Whole Person

As part of the AHMA, I learned about the "whole person" approach to medicine: body, mind, and spirit. After much studying and careful, patient monitoring, it became apparent to me that the causes of disease often come from within, rather than from external sources. Until I fully comprehended this, I could not completely heal, nor could the patient be considered completely healthy. I learned that the entire body was a totally synchronized energy machine; if there were a restriction of energy in a specific region of the body, weakness or breakdown in that area could ultimately occur.

❧ Emotions Translate into the Physical

When I began to study patterns in patients, I finally understood more about the true causes of disease and health. The emotions, such as fear, anger, hatred, jealousy, envy, and prejudices, kill the spirit and hence the very nature of man. The person who is filled with emotions such as these is sick physically, mentally, and spiritually. For example, patients who were more fixed in their thought and behavior patterns often suffered from arthritis. Rigidity in thoughts created inflexibility in the body. Persons who had pent-up emotions and were under a lot of stress frequently had hypertension, which is indeed unrelieved internal pressure. Interestingly enough, these types of patients seldom developed cancer, which seemed to be caused by other types of behavior, such as fear of loss or loneliness. Often patients who had difficulty expressing love and other personal feelings had blocked coronary (heart) arteries. At times, these patients may have felt unloved as well.

Applying these concepts to the other diseases of modern society, we find that AIDS is "Anger Internally Directed at Self." The whole category of immune suppression diseases has to do with a host of issues directed inwardly at the patient's life-force. This creates disturbances of the immune system. We know that immune suppression is regulated by a part of the brain called the hypothalamus. It helps to modulate emotions such as joy, happiness, sadness, and anger. We understand that our environment is full of toxins and poisons.

However, it is obvious that simply being exposed to these poisonous substances does not necessarily mean that disease will prevail.

Repeatedly we physicians see two people in the same family who are subjected to similar problems yet may have completely different responses. One may have a disease; the other may be totally healthy. Generally the difference lies in their individual attitudes and behaviors. So many problems are the result of the inability to release old, suppressed hurts of the past. It is these hurts that intrude from the subconscious as reminders of some perceived injury. This injury lodges in the region of the body that most appropriately relates to the emotion. For instance, love has to do with the heart, breast, or bladder, which are the giving glands.

Time and time again we are told to give up the old hurts and negative emotions. If we do not do this, they could clearly manifest as disease or injury. The body literally starts "taking it out on itself."

❦ THE HEALING POWER OF LOVE

On the positive side of health, love is the purest and most important emotion that we can express. Love, taken to its highest form, is the most profound expression of our spiritual selves. At this elevated creation love is called unconditional by some religions while other religions refer to this as "agape." Here we love fully, no matter what happens—no "ifs," "ands," or "buts." When love is openly given to others miracles can happen.

There is a complete lack of judgment here. We know judgment of others, as well as self, can limit health and healing and create blocks of negative emotion. Anger, fear, and guilt are some of the most destructive emotions. These cause blocks in the natural energy flow of the body that could ultimately lead to breakdown and disease. The opposite of this is love and the expression of it. Love is the most healing modality known on earth today.

❦ REMOVING BLOCKS

What is the key for diagnosing and releasing these patterns? One effective procedure is hypnotherapy. In competent hands this process can remove deep blocks. Once these blocks are removed healing can occur.

Hypnosis is a profound and safe way to connect with the deep inner self, sometimes called the subconscious or even the superconscious. This part of us is very powerful and contains much data that is helpful. Often, by tapping into this portion of ourselves, we may achieve amazing results with our health.

There are many physical reasons for a breakdown, such as hereditary weakness, nutritional deficiency, fatigue, and accidents. But they often are linked to a deeper pattern. There is a positive effect from simply seeing the problem; that is, digging it out of the subconscious and experiencing it at a pleasurable, conscious level. Releasing the problem will likely cause the physical condition to disappear eventually. Simple as this seems, it works. Similar changes occur with homeopathic remedies, particularly if they are high dilutions. If the right remedy is given they help to remove the negative emotion.

Obviously each person must deal with many emotions. Removing these problems one at a time is like peeling away multiple layers of onion skins. They unfold, one at a time, until you get down to the sweet, internal part. This healthy, inner core is vibrant and complete within itself, free of illness.

You have the freedom to change negative emotions any time you want. But always do it with joy. Joy is not only a result of achieving this balanced center, but a joyful attitude along the way helps the process of finding that new inner peace as well.

🦋 HUMAN POTENTIAL DEVELOPMENT SCALE

Throughout history, philosophers and religious leaders have emphasized that there are certain characteristics that represent the highest potential for service to and interaction with humanity. There is no test that we know of that measures this development, although the Human Potential Attitude Inventory gives you some hints. I would like to offer you here an opportunity to measure your feelings about your development at this point in time. I suggest you take the following test in your ordinary state of consciousness, just by reading it. Then get into a deep state of relaxation, ask yourself the same questions, and rate yourself from that point of view. Zero means total lack of the quality; 100 implies the maximum any person could possibly achieve.

This is a self-assessment test. It will help you determine your level of attainment of some of the attributes we most aspire to.

HUMAN POTENTIAL DEVELOPMENT

Love	0 5 10 15 20 25 30 35 40 45 50 55 60 65 70 75 80 85 90 95 100
Wisdom	0 5 10 15 20 25 30 35 40 45 50 55 60 65 70 75 80 85 90 95 100
Will	0 5 10 15 20 25 30 35 40 45 50 55 60 65 70 75 80 85 90 95 100
Faith	0 5 10 15 20 25 30 35 40 45 50 55 60 65 70 75 80 85 90 95 100
Hope	0 5 10 15 20 25 30 35 40 45 50 55 60 65 70 75 80 85 90 95 100
Charity	0 5 10 15 20 25 30 35 40 45 50 55 60 65 70 75 80 85 90 95 100
Courage	0 5 10 15 20 25 30 35 40 45 50 55 60 65 70 75 80 85 90 95 100
Joy	0 5 10 15 20 25 30 35 40 45 50 55 60 65 70 75 80 85 90 95 100
Motivation	0 5 10 15 20 25 30 35 40 45 50 55 60 65 70 75 80 85 90 95 100
Confidence	0 5 10 15 20 25 30 35 40 45 50 55 60 65 70 75 80 85 90 95 100
Compassion	0 5 10 15 20 25 30 35 40 45 50 55 60 65 70 75 80 85 90 95 100
Serenity	0 5 10 15 20 25 30 35 40 45 50 55 60 65 70 75 80 85 90 95 100
Tolerance	0 5 10 15 20 25 30 35 40 45 50 55 60 65 70 75 80 85 90 95 100
Forgiveness	0 5 10 15 20 25 30 35 40 45 50 55 60 65 70 75 80 85 90 95 100

CHAPTER 3

Holistic Medicine and Hidden Disease

HOLISTIC PHILOSOPHY

HOLISTIC MEDICINE REPRESENTS a philosophy of looking at all aspects of the individual and using multiple methods to effect positive results for better health, happiness, and improved life-style functioning. As a system, holistic medicine considers body, mind, and spirit. It looks profoundly into the causes of illness.

THE ILLNESS SPECTRUM

IN SOME WAYS we recognize that there is a continuum between being only slightly out of balance and being seriously ill and bedridden. At one end of the scale the seriousness of the condition is readily apparent at times; at the beginning the condition may appear more subtle. The significance of this is that there may be mild symptoms such as fatigue, headaches, aches and pains, and temporary thought disturbances at certain stages of diseases.

While these symptoms may interfere dramatically with the individual's life-style and ability to function, they may not be given credibility or diagnosed by professionals. These subtle symptoms are largely ignored by the average physician who is more accustomed to dealing with crisis situations in medicine.

Insurance companies and the medical profession want firm, black-and-white diagnoses with cut-and-dried treatments. In the holistic view most illnesses, except for accidents, take years to develop. An example is atherosclerosis, in which the formation of plaques in the arteries slowly interrupts the blood supply to vital organs, which may take a long time to build up. Abuse of the digestive system and pancreas by excessive intake of sugar and fats until diabetes or liver problems occur is another common example.

❧ Subtle Diseases

Consequently, a disease may begin with mild signs and symptoms and after years may develop into a life-threatening situation. Alternately, the disease may be mild and continue as an annoyance to the patient for a long time without getting worse or ever significantly improving. Therefore, it may continue as a chronic, longstanding disruption to the patient's performance and general well being. I label these problems the "subtle diseases" of our modern society.

Chronic Fatigue and Immune Dysfunction Syndrome
An example is the Chronic Fatigue and Immune Dysfunction Syndrome. Until the last several years it was largely ignored by the general medical profession and governmental agencies. Yet it affects thousands of people profoundly, incapacitating many of them. Only recently did the U.S. Center of Disease Control officially classify it as a real disease.

Yeast Infections
Another problem is yeast infections, specifically called *Candidiasis*, a fungus. This controversial problem has grown in the last few years because of increased use of antibiotics and steroids. Both medications promote the abundant overgrowth of the fungus *Candida Albicans*. Children frequently get this infection in their oral cavities, resulting in a condition called "thrush." Women experience a frustrating and annoying vaginitis or vaginal infection caused by this organism. It may be recurrent, causing multiple infections throughout the indi-

vidual's lifetime. The fungus can attack many organs and cause systemic problems as well.

Some physicians claim there is no real disease here, yet I have personally seen many patients improve once this fungus is treated and removed. A recent study revealed that many cases of premenstrual syndrome (PMS) improved once *Candidiasis* was adequately treated.

Tinnitus

Tinnitus is the perception of abnormal ear or head noises. People often complain of a constant or intermittent buzzing or ringing in the ears. At times it is persistent and may be associated with hearing loss. It may interfere with the ability to concentrate and sleep and may prevent a normal life-style.

Allopathic medicine really offers no successful treatment for this annoying disease. On the other hand, I have recently developed a program that has created success in some people. I use an electrical stimulating device, applied directly to the ear; homeopathic injections, called mucokehl. I recommend injections of the D5 strength —½ cc with ¼ cc of 1 percent procaine injected intradermally, behind the ear over the mastoid bone. I use 8 injections—2 per week for 4 weeks. These injections immediately follow the electrical stimulation treatment—and should be done on the same day.

I also recommend taking the herb gingko biloba—250 mg twice daily.

Every other day I administer two drops of the essential oil helichrysum placed on the tips of the index finger and inserted into the ear canal. Another drop is applied over the mastoid bone behind the ear. If this therapy is administered simultaneously with the homeopathic treatment, the treatments should occur on alternate days.

Finally, dairy products—specifically cheese—should be eliminated from the diet.

If after applying these modalities the tinnitus still persists, then I include a series of chelation treatments (see Chapter 9).

I have had success with this therapy, in some cases completely eliminating the buzzing and in others reducing the annoying sounds to a more tolerable level. Be aware that this is a completely safe treatment and that the medical profession as a whole has nothing to offer the sufferers of tinnitus.

The real attributes of a holistic physician lie in taking the time to care for patients by listening intently to their complaints and delving deeply in order to find the cause of their problems. We physicians have to be more attentive and "practice the art" as well as the science of medicine as our forbears intended us to do.

CHAPTER 4

The True Cause of Disease and Wellness

TRUE HEALTH

TRUE HEALTH IS A BALANCE of the three aspects of the human being: body, mind, and spirit. In the holistic approach, we consider the mind as the electrical control center. It sends thoughts out into the environment as well as triggering electrical impulses that travel throughout the body. It controls organs, muscles, and glands, as well as the spirit, the life force that energizes as well as unites and otherwise forms a cohesiveness of the body and mind. When all of the parts are operating smoothly, there is a balance and a healthy, vital, active person.

When any one of these aspects is out of balance there is a breakdown. How does an imbalance occur? If the body is diseased, then it will begin to deteriorate. If there are improper or destructive thoughts, such as hate, malice, selfishness, and covetousness, then improper messages are sent out and are reflected back to the sender, causing disorder and disease. What you send out you get back! When the spirit — or life force — is weak, then the body and/or mind malfunctions and degeneration occurs.

Several years ago, while attempting to awaken public interest in the enormous problems in the health of the peoples of the world, the director of the World Health Organization made a profound statement. He said, "Major strides will only be made in world health when we finally realize that good health is much more than the absence of disease." We should strive for a high level of health and wellness, he said. Our minds need to be clear to think and reason with inspiration.

Our health represents a mirror of our life path and the flow of vitality while traveling it! If a part of the whole is over-stressed, uneasy, out-of-ease, or "dis-eased," then the whole body feels it; thus, a total body approach is the answer.

🌿 HEALTH IS LIKE A SCALE

Homeostasis is described as a state of equilibrium or balance of the body environment. There are new ways of looking at homeostasis, including new parameters with which to measure it. This includes the use of entirely new tools as well as new interpretations of the old tools consisting of blood, urine, and tissue chemistries. A good descriptive model for explaining homeostasis is a scale. On one side there are factors that cause breakdown or degeneration of the body, and on the other side are factors that build or regenerate the body. Once it is understood that the body chemistry must be in balance, like a scale, then those elements that affect the process must be identified.

Generally speaking the three primary factors affecting the body parameters are diet, structure, and emotions. When any or all of these are operating in an excessively stressful manner, change occurs at the molecular or biochemical level. If this process is prolonged and extensive, then changes occur on the physical level and signs and symptoms of disease begin to appear. The process from the initial biochemical imbalance to total disease and breakdown may take months or even years. All during this time the body is attempting to fight off infection, repair the body systems, and reestablish balance, or homeostasis.

Let's see first how this works at the biochemical level. The description revolves around a very simple principle that is understood by few and applied by even fewer. Simply stated the principle is: the workhorses of the human body are enzymes, coenzymes, and hormones. The effective molecular structure of these biochemical products depends upon functioning minerals.

"Functioning" is the key word. What determines if a mineral is functioning? Is it getting the job done? One minor and two major factors must be considered. The minor factor is the occurrence of a real deficiency of a mineral in the body. The two major factors are:

1. A deficiency produced by an inhibited function; and
2. A toxicity of one mineral to another, resulting from the consistent presence of the nonfunctioning mineral. To function properly minerals must be in a proper ratio to each other.

Referring to the model of the scale (see figure 4-1), the more destructive factors are placed on one side of the scale, the more it tilts to that side. The body attempts to compensate with many mechanisms. If it fails, the scale tips over completely and we may experience disease. We hope, though, that the body mechanisms of homeostasis, with the help of external adjunctive therapy, will produce balance and health.

It is easy to see how state of balance can be a matter of degree. On one side of the scale there is degeneration, and on the other, there is regeneration. Naturally, the body cells that make up organs eventually age and die, only to be replaced by new cells. This process may be accelerated by injury, lack of good nutrition, and the presence of assaulting substances such as heavy metals that include lead and mercury. These metals, when picked up by the cells, accelerate the aging process. This process is called "cellular oxidation."

There are substances called anti-oxidants that block the effects of the heavy metals and the premature aging process. Anti-oxidants are generally considered to be vitamins A, C, E and the trace element selenium. They are easy to remember; think ACES.

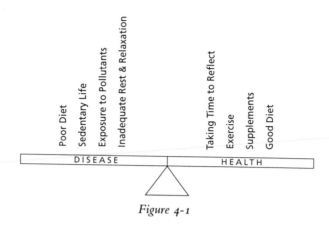

Figure 4-1

A new study reveals that people who are healthy in their old age have a large amount of glutathione, another powerful anti-oxidant, in their bodies. This protein apparently protects them from toxins and other destructive chemicals, ultimately leading to healthy longevity.

It is not known whether these individuals assimilate and accumulate more of the product glutathione or whether they utilize more and hence have less in storage. Some of the reasons for utilizing more glutathione is that certain persons may be exposed to more toxins in their environment.

Degeneration occurs when the breakdown of body tissue occurs faster than the repair or rebuilding. Conversely, when repair and regrowth of tissue is more rapid than destruction, regeneration occurs. According to recent reports, an average person is generally in a regenerative phase until approximately twenty-eight years of age. At this time, a neutral point is reached at which degeneration and regeneration occur at about the same rate. After this time, degeneration occurs faster than regeneration, unless healthy steps are taken. Functioning and nonfunctioning of minerals is measured by interpreting the mineral ratio in blood and tissue tests.

The previously mentioned three broad areas of one's chosen life-style—diet, structure, and emotions—either inhibit or enhance homeostasis through the mineral ratios, one to another, working through the endocrine glands. The endocrine glands can be defined as miniature factories that produce and release internal chemical hormones that regulate many body processes.

Measuring the Body's Electromagnetic Field

Recently a nuclear magnetic resonance machine, or N.M.R., has been utilized to measure the disturbance of the electromagnetic energy field that is found around all living things. It can measure the smallest component including details of the individual cells. This energy reflects, in a manner of speaking, the life-force of a substance. Incredibly, the N.M.R is able to detect electromagnetic changes in the body as early as one year prior to the establishment of cancer cells. Consequently we now have an early precancer detection tool, which, very importantly, is also completely safe, and has no side effects.

This energy can also be photographed with a process called Kirlian photography, by which parts of the body, generally the fingers or toes, are placed between two electrically charged magnetic plates and photographed. An energy field is observed and measured around these extremities. The force of the field is a reflection of the strength of the persons' vital life-force.

The problems that could occur in each of the three areas are:

1. Food and drink that upset the mineral ratio are ingested;
2. Significant unattended structural problems drain energy; and
3. Emotions that prevent enjoyment in the now are chosen.

Generally speaking, there are other very important factors in our life-style to be considered. Exercise is critical to good health. It improves circulation, digestive functions, muscle tone, and bone density, preserving the strength of bones. If exercise is performed regularly and adequately, it produces internal hormones that heal. These are called endorphins. Endorphins can even block any pain one might be experiencing.

Another factor to be considered is the air you breath. Are there poisonous gases and toxins, such as pesticides, present? These could be, and probably are, detrimental to the body when inhaled and accumulated.

Are you receiving these same toxins in your diet? Again, while small portions may not harm you, daily ingestion of these unwanted substances over long periods of time may build up. These high doses accumulated in the body can eventually cause disease.

Do you smoke? If you do you are directly exposing yourself to tar, nicotine, and carbon monoxide. The later is the same gas that is expelled from automobiles. Carbon monoxide competes with our circulating oxygen levels, depleting the amounts available to our brains, muscles, and other organs.

Alcohol has very few nutrients in it and consequently is considered empty calories, breaking down into sugar. It lacks the enzymes, coenzymes, and other vitamins and minerals necessary to support the body. Also some of the additives involved in the production of alcohol could have side effects.

Studies have been done on the prolonged watching of television. When one considers the amount of scary news that is being shown, one can't help but think of the stress it can cause. One study performed several years ago in Miami demonstrated that most people experience a rise in blood pressure after watching television for four to five hours daily.

Working can be stressful, particularly if you are subjected to certain pressures. Fumes, dust, loud noises, and fluorescent lights all cause stress and imbalance in our bodies. Irregular or long hours and particularly night shifts seem to create an imbalance in our own natural body rhythms. It has been shown that darkness during sleep, without the influence of the sun's rays, allows the body to renew and regenerate. Tests show that people working the night shift have greater problems with their emotions and immune systems. This may reflect the fact that the pineal gland, which naturally secretes the hormone melatonin, is influenced by the sun's radiation waves. Also artificial lighting may cause more agitation and the inability to concentrate. Dr. John Ott did much research on a process called full spectrum lighting, meaning light that contains all of the colors of white light when refracted by a prism. He worked with subjects in the military and from the public school systems. When schoolrooms were converted from fluorescent lighting to full spectrum lighting, in some cases the grade point average of the students went up by at least one grade. In most cases their agitation and fidgeting, as recorded by time-lapse cameras, diminished.

One other very important way to combat stress is to make a commitment to relax during the day. If one is able to take some quiet time, to rest or meditate, apparently regeneration and renewal occurs. Remember the phrase: "Prayer is talking to God and meditation is listening to his answers."

However, remember that after passing the age of twenty-eight, degeneration is in the driver's seat. To avert this, we must take steps to prevent the intervention of harmful, stressful factors from adversely affecting us. Thus, we may choose to take more vitamins and minerals, improve our diet, get more exercise, take more time to reflect, and achieve other good health habits. In doing these things we may stall the aging process. (For more on this subject, see Chapter 22.)

In order to help you assess your stress level, I have included a "Personal Stress Assessment Test" at the end of this chapter.

⚸ Model of Wellness

I have defined disease fairly thoroughly by now. However, it is important to think in terms of the body being out-of-ease with itself, or "dis-eased." We must think of disease as a process rather than a static state or the result of an end stage of the degeneration process. Healing is an on-going process as well. There are degrees of wellness and illness. Disease, at the opposite end of the scale from health, is a manifestation of illness or lack of wellness. There is a constant effort by the body mechanisms, including blood and lymph circulation, immune, digestive, and hormone systems, and others, to bring the body into a balanced or a homeostatic condition. In this condition an individual has no apparent signs or symptoms of disease.

Wellness, then, is more than a lack of illness or disease; it is a feeling of well being. It is the ability to regenerate the cells and tissues toward a healthy, viable state. It is the capacity to function more and at a higher level. Taken to its ultimate definition, it is the ability to create those things that are best for our soul growth. It is total alignment and harmony of the four bodies (aspects of ourselves): mental, physical, emotional, and spiritual. It is the capacity to manifest the ideal situation for you, whatever that may be.

Dr. John Travis's "Model of Wellness" is helpful in understanding this process.

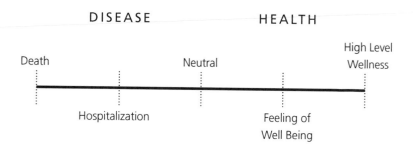

DYNAMIC SCALE OF DISEASE AND HEALTH

In the middle, there is a neutral point where a person is just surviving, not fully well nor really ill. On one end, there is disease, that represents disability, hospitalization, and possibly an end stage, or death. On the opposite end, there is high-level wellness, in which the body may be functioning at the highest level as mentioned earlier. In between are levels of illness and wellness.

After viewing the cause of disease and illness it should be apparent that there is a new medical model, a new way of looking at health or the lack of it. Our goals should be to achieve balance in the four aspects of ourselves—the body, the mind, the emotions, and the spirit—leading us to function at a highly evolved level, experiencing joy and happiness and relating in a balanced manner to our environment. This should enable us to be creative and thus evolve into the highest ideal of the person we want to be.

REFERENCES:

Ott, John N. *Health and Light: The Effects of Natural and Artificial Light on Man and Other Living Things*. New York: Pocket Books, 1976.

PERSONAL STRESS ASSESSMENT
Total Life Stress Test ⋆

Take the Total Life Stress Test and begin to see what you need to do to reduce stress in your life. Record your stress points on the lines in the right-hand margin, and indicate subtotals on the lines at the end of each subsection. Subtotal your stress points at the end of each section. Then add your subtotals to determine your total score.

I. CHEMICAL STRESS

A. DIETARY STRESS	Scoring	Points
Average Daily Sugar Consumption:		
Sugar added to food or drink	1 pt. per 5 tsp	____
Sweet roll, piece of pie/cake, brownie, other desert	1 point ea.	____
Coke or can of pop, candy bar	2 points ea.	____
Banana split, commercial milk shake, sundae, etc.	5 points ea.	____
White flour (white bread, spaghetti, etc.)	5 points	____
Average Daily Salt Consumption:		
Little or no "added" salt	0 points	____
Few salty foods (pretzels, potato chips, etc.)	0 points	____
Moderate "added" salt and/or salty foods at least once per day	3 points	____
Heavy salt user (use of "table salt" and/or salty foods at least twice per day	10 points	____
Average Daily Caffeine Consumption:		
Coffee	½ pt. ea. cup	____
Tea	½ pt. ea. cup	____
Cola drink or Mountain Dew	1 pt. ea. cup	____
2 Anacin or APC tabs	½ pt. per dose	____
Caffeine Benzoate tablets (NoDoz, Vivarin, etc.)	2 points ea.	____
Dietary Stress Subtotal:		____

B. OTHER CHEMICAL STRESS

	Scoring	Points
Drinking Water:		
Chlorinated only	1 point	_____
Chlorinated and Fluoridated	2 points	_____
Soil and Air Pollution:		
Live within 10 miles of city of 500,000 or more	10 points	_____
Live within 10 miles of city of 250,000 or more	5 points	_____
Live within 10 miles of city of 50,000 or more	2 points	_____
Live in the country but use pesticides, herbicides and/or chemical fertilizer	10 points	_____
Exposed to cigarette smoke of someone else more than one hour per day	5 points	_____
Drugs (any amount of usage):		
Antidepressants	1 point	_____
Tranquilizers	3 points	_____
Sleeping pills	3 points	_____
Narcotics	5 points	_____
Other pain relievers	3 points	_____
Nicotine:		
3-10 cigarettes per day	5 points	_____
11-20 cigarettes per day	15 points	_____
21-30 cigarettes per day	20 points	_____
31-40 cigarettes per day	35 points	_____
Over 40 cigarettes per day	40 points	_____
Cigar(s) per day	1 point ea	_____
Pipeful(s) of tobacco per day	1 point ea.	_____
Chewing tobacco — "chews" per day	1 point ea.	_____

★ Adapted from *The Stress Connection* by C. Norman Shealy, M.D. Springfield, MO (1993). Reproduced with permission of the author and publisher.

Average Daily Alcohol Consumption:		Points
1 oz. whiskey, gin vodka, etc.	2 points ea	_____
8 oz. beer	2 points ea.	_____
4-6 oz. glass of wine	2 points ea	_____

Other Chemical Stress Subtotal: _____

Chemical Stress Total: _____

II. PHYSICAL STRESS

Weight:

Underweight more than 10 lbs.	5 points	_____
10 to 15 lbs overweight	5 points	_____
16 to 25 lbs overweight	10 points	_____
26 to 40 lbs overweight	25 points	_____
More than 40 lbs overweight	40 points	_____

Activity:

Adequate exercise**, 2+ days per week	0 points	_____
Some physical exercise, 1 or 2 days per week	15 points	_____
No regular exercise	40 points	_____

Work Stress:

Sit most of the day	3 points	_____
Industrial/factory worker	3 points	_____
Overnight travel more than once a week	5 points	_____
Work more than 50 hours per week	2 pts. per hour over 50 hours	_____
Work varying shifts	10 points	_____
Work night shift	5 points	_____
Heavy labor - physically fit	0 points	_____
Heavy labor - not physically fit	40 points	_____

Physical Stress Total: _____

** Adequate exercise means doubling heartbeat and/or sweating a minimum of 30 minutes per time.

III. ATTITUDINAL STRESS

A. HOLMES-RAHE SOCIAL READJUSTMENT RATING***

Circle the values that correspond with the life events listed below that you have experienced during the past twelve months.

Death of a spouse 100
Divorce 73
Marital separation 65
Jail term 63
Death of a close family member 63
Personal injury or illness 53
Marriage 50
Fired at work 47
Marital reconciliation 45
Retirement 45
Change in the health of family member 44
Pregnancy 40
Sexual difficulties 39
Gain of new family member 39
Business readjustment 39
Change in financial state 38
Death of close friend 37
Change to a different line of work 36
Change in the number of arguments with spouse 35
Mortgage over $20,000 31
Foreclosure of mortgage or loan 30
Change in responsibilities at work 29
Son or daughter leaving home 29
Trouble with in-laws 29
Outstanding personal achievement 28
Spouse beginning or stopping work 26
Beginning or ending school 25
Change in living conditions 24

***Adapted from Holmes, T.H. and R.H. Rahe. "The Social Readjustment Rating Scale," from *Journal of Psychosomatic Research*, 11 (1967): 213-218. Reproduced with permission of the authors and publisher.

Revision of personal habits 23
Trouble with boss 20
Change in work hours or conditions 20
Change in residence 20
Change in schools 19
Change in recreation 19
Change in church activities 18
Change in social activities 17
Mortgage or loan less than $20,000 16
Change in sleeping habits 15
Change in eating habits 15
Vacation, especially if away from home 13
Christmas, or other major holiday stress 12
Minor violations of the law 11

Holmes-Rahe Social Readjustment Total: _____

Add the values to get the Holmes-Rahe Social Readjustment total. Then refer to the conversion table below to determine your number of Life Stress points.

CONVERSION TABLE

HOLMES-RAHE less than	Your number of points	HOLMES-RAHE less than	Your number of points
60	0	280	16
110	1	285	17
160	2	290	18
170	3	295	19
180	4	300	20
190	5	305	21
200	6	310	22
210	7	315	23
220	8	320	24
230	9	325	25
240	10	330	26
250	11	335	27
260	12	340	28
265	13	345	29
270	14	350	30
275	15	Over 350	40

Holmes-Rahe Stress Point Total (converted): . . . . _____

B. OTHER EMOTIONAL STRESS

		Points
Sleep:		
Less than 7 hours per night	3 points	_____
Usually 7 or 8 hours per night	0 points	_____
More than 8 hours per night	2 points	_____
Relaxation:		
Relax only during sleep	10 points	_____
Relax or meditate at least 20 minutes per day	0 points	_____
Frustration at Work:		
Enjoy work	0 points	_____
Mildly frustrated by job	1 point	_____
Moderately frustrated by job	3 points	_____
Very frustrated by job	5 point	_____
Lack of authority job	5 points	_____
Boss doesn't trust me	5 points	_____
Marital Status:		
Married, happily	0 points	_____
Married, moderately unhappy	2 points	_____
Married, very unhappy	5 points	_____
Unmarried man over 30	5 points	_____
Unmarried woman over 30	2 points	_____
Usual Mood:		
Happy, well adjusted	0 points	_____
Moderately angry, depressed or frustrated	10 points	_____
Very angry, depressed or frustrated	20 points	_____
Overall Attitude:		
Hopeless	10-40 points	_____
Depressed	10-40 points	_____
Unable to achieve major goal	10-40 points	_____
Unable to achieve close love/intimacy	10-40 points	_____
Frustrated, annoyed, and/or angry because someone attacked or harmed me or prevented me from happiness	10-40 points	_____
Satisfied and in control of my life	0 points	_____

		Points
Experience happiness regularly	0 points	_____
Believe I am responsible for my happiness	0 points	_____
Believe happiness is an inside job	0 points	_____
Any other major emotional stress not mentioned above (You judge intensity)	10-40 points	_____

Attitudinal Stress Total: _____

Total Life Stress

I.   Chemical Stress Total: _____

II. Physical Stress Total: _____

III. Attitudinal Stress Total: _____

TOTAL LIFE STRESS SCORE: _____

If your total score exceeds 24 points, you will probably feel better if you reduce your stress; greater than 50 points, you definitely need to eliminate stress in your life.

Circle your stressor with the highest number of points and work first to eliminate it; then circle your next greatest stressor, overcome it; and so on.

Now look at some of the ways your body may react to stress. Please be aware that if you have any major or worrisome symptoms, or more than fifteen total symptoms, you should consult your physician before deciding that stress is the cause of your symptoms.

CHAPTER 5

Disease (Being Out-of-Ease with Self)

DISEASES OUT OF CONTROL

WE ARE ENTERING very interesting times, times of change and times of challenge. While this is true in all walks of life, it is particularly true in the field of medicine. While I am honored to be a founding member and a past ruling board member of the American Holistic Medical Association, I am also pleased to be a member of the Arizona Homeopathic Medical Association. These two organizations are similar, one operating internationally and the other on a state level. Their initials are the same, A.H.M.A. Both share the common denominator of encouraging education and complementary medicine.

ASSAULT ON THE IMMUNE SYSTEM

There is much frustration on the part of the two partners in health care, the patient and the physician, as a consequence of two major factors. One is the explosion of diseases that principally involve the immune system. These include AIDS and Epstein-Barr Syndrome or, as it is more recently called, Chronic Fatigue and Immune Dysfunction Syndrome. Also added to this list are diseases such as arthritis, food allergies, candidiasis (yeast infections), and severe environmental sensitivities. All have a common denominator: an immune system that has been injured by constant subjection to an environment containing stressors that are hazardous to the body. This is exaggerated by prolonged and constant exposure to toxins, such as pesticides, chemical preservatives, antibiotics, and heavy metals. Electromagnetic pollution can also be a problem.

HEALTH CARE COSTS OUT OF CONTROL

The second factor is the rising cost of health care in the United States, which was $300 billion in 1977 and is reportedly now over $1 trillion annually.

A NEW PARADIGM

These major issues have forced many of my colleagues and me to rethink our present approach to medicine. At the same time the government has been issuing statements revealing the new direction of health care in the United States.

There is much talk concerning a "paradigm shift" of the future, where old truths that we consider guides to rule our lives no longer work for us and new truths are to be accepted. Surprisingly, all these predictions are coming true; we are in the future and all are a part of its manifestation. A new type of medicine in which we rely more on natural modalities to cure illnesses is becoming popular.

I attended an AHMA medical retreat in which we not only dealt with national organizational issues, but also dealt with personal issues such as codependency and personal growth. As the physicians and health-care providers at the retreat began to share personal experiences, we observed that many of us were facing similar problems, although our process for healing was perhaps different. Once we had gone through the toughest challenges of our lives, those being struggles with our own deepest fears, our focus became clear. Then, and only then, could we be effective in helping others. We had gone through a shift in personal consciousness. We learned that incurable diseases, such as amyotrophic lateral sclerosis, multiple sclerosis, and heart disease, are being cured. Interestingly, in these cases, a change in consciousness usually preceded or was observed concurrently with the physical healing.

Many of the individuals attending the retreat claimed they had experienced a frustrating and painful childhood and carried these scars into adulthood without even being fully aware of the personality interaction. However, it is not necessary to carry this burden forever. Our board president, Dr. Bernie Siegel, author of the best-selling book *Love, Medicine, and Miracles* (Harper and Row, 1986) said, "It is never too late to have a good childhood." This meant to me that we won't have to continue to live with our fears, hurts, and other scars but can eliminate them—sort of relive our childhood in a pleasant way. This can be assisted by using proven techniques such as one-on-one or group support therapy, visualization, and hypnosis. After the health-care provider goes through this process, he, too, can become an effective support system. He can become a role model for people who have chosen to experience sickness or disease or, as I refer to it, "being out-of-ease" with self and one's surroundings.

✄ TRANSITION AND ACCELERATION

Once these areas are dealt with, the appropriate use of nutrition, herbs, homeopathic remedies, aromatherapy, vitamins, and minerals can aid in bringing rapid healing to the body. It also appears now that today everything is accelerated and diseases that originally needed years of therapy to heal can be reversed in months or even weeks.

Yes, things truly are changing right before our very eyes. In fact, last year 30 percent of health-care visits to professionals were to persons practising alternatiuve therapies. But all of us can be a part of this process instead of being on the outside looking in, too fearful to get involved. Now is the time to take personal responsibility and visualize healing our selves, our families, our friends, and even our planet.

Section Two

DISEASES AND THERAPIES
OF THE TWENTY-FIRST CENTURY

IN THIS SECTION I introduce the more common diseases and conditions that we see today in medicine. These are diseases of great concern, for they are responsible for most of the death, disability, and suffering in our society today.

I reveal how they may be identified and diagnosed. I have included some very valuable questionnaires to help you identify whether a disease is present in you and, if so, how it can be treated.

Most important is that I present therapies that are, in some cases, innovative but are not taught to the average physician in medical school in the United States. They are also therapies that are utilized in other countries and are found in historical medical references and are proven to be safe and effective. These therapies may at times be able to reverse a disease that has been pronounced incurable by other medical authorities. If this is giving hope when hope was lost, then that in itself is very valuable.

CHAPTER 6

Alternative Health Care

THE ALTERNATIVES

THERE ARE A NUMBER of modalities used in complementary (alternative) medicine. Several are described in this chapter—homeopathy, herbal therapy, acupuncture, and manipulation of the body—while I have devoted individual chapters to others, such as chelation, aromatherapy, and cleansing. Others, such as nutrition, diet, dietary supplements, visualization, hypnotherapy, aromatherapy, allopathic medicine, and other therapies, are described throughout this book as they apply to a given problem or disease.

🥀 HOMEOPATHY

History of Homeopathy
During the 1700s and 1800s the predominant mode of health care practiced in the United States was a philosophy called "homeopathy." This discipline was based on the belief that healing must first come from within, accompanied by divine guidance. Through the years it was also believed that the body inherently knew what was good for it and that if given adequate elements of herbs, vitamins, minerals, and all other nutrients, it would properly use them to maintain health.

Homeopathic Medicine

It was further thought that if a substance created symptoms, then minute doses of this same or a like substance would reverse the symptoms and effect a cure. Furthermore, it was found that the more diluted or weaker the substance was, the more powerful was the effect. When I visited Thomas Jefferson's restored family home, Monticello, in Virginia, I observed a homeopathic kit in the study that reportedly belonged to this great gentleman.

Later, when the germ theory was formulated, medicine began looking for stronger substances to kill the germs, creating a medical science called "allopathy," the medical philosophy most prevalent in the United States today. Unfortunately, this philosophy largely ignores one's personal resistance and immunity to disease. For instance, two people may be exposed to the same germ but only one person gets the disease.

Pharmaceutical companies encouraged the growth of allopathic medicine because they could see the possibility of profits in the production and sales of many kinds of drugs. Consequently, an inadequately informed public and lack of financial backing caused homeopathic schools to be phased out in the early 1900s.

Other countries still use homeopathy as the primary line of defense. The personal physician of the Queen Mother of England is a homeopath, for example. The Queen Mother is now well over ninety years of age and is doing well with this medicine.

Germ-warfare

During the last seventy to eighty years medicine has seen what many physicians call the contra-casual approach—the germ theory, based on the concept that germs are inherently bad and we must concentrate on destroying them. This approach has led to all the chemotherapeutic interventions that are so much a part of mainstream medicine today.

At this time, germ-warfare is proving less than effective against immune disorders. Additionally, the side effects from pharmaceuticals have contributed to a virtual epidemic of iatrogenic ills—that is, adverse conditions actually induced by medical treatment, at a cost of $77 billion per year. Sadly, the pharmaceutical industry has much at stake in continuing to promote the use of sophisticated chemicals even though they are very often detrimental to our basic biological makeup.

Our escalating health problems are forcing researchers to explore new means of not merely treating new diseases, but bolstering our resistance to all types of ailments.

Nature Works

The philosophy of using herbs, essential oils, and homeopathic remedies and working with forces of nature fell into disrepute in the early 1900s. Instead, resources that pretended to control nature and manipulate the human body into adaptation were mobilized. For instance, instead of properly caring for the body, the divine vessel of the soul, with nutrients, we generally either abuse or ignore it and therefore create much disease or imbalance, and at times, premature death.

❀ HERBAL THERAPY

Herbs are very potent healers. After all, many of our medicines are derived from herbs. Diseases can be manipulated by the therapeutic use of herbs. While the United States has lagged behind, much of the rest of the world has relied largely on homeopathic remedies, herbs, and other natural healing techniques. Dr. Steven Ross, director of the World Health Research Organization, told this story when he returned from China where he exchanged medical information. A Chinese doctor asked Dr. Ross how alternative medical therapies were faring in the United States. He replied that homeopathy and herbal therapy were not too popular, to which the Chinese doctor said, "No, I don't mean that. I mean the use of drugs and surgery. Don't forget, we have used acupuncture and herbs for more than 5,000 years and we know the results of every combination as well as when and where to use these products."

In contrast, he pointed out, many American surgical techniques are still experimental and many drugs have been tested only for a few years. Consequently, little or nothing is known about their combinations or long-term side effects on the body. The Chinese doctor considered these therapies to be experimental.

༄ ACUPUNCTURE

Acupuncture is a therapy whereby one applies needles, pressure, and laser burning or electricity to the skin to effect positive changes in organs of the body or to abolish pain.

History of Acupuncture

Acupuncture has been used for 5,000 years in China, perhaps making it the world's oldest system of healing. In the 1700s, Jesuit priests from France, after learning of the miracles of acupuncture in their travels to China, brought this therapy back home to Europe. Later, excavation of an old Chinese city uncovered what was termed "The Yellow Emperor's Canon of Internal Medicine"—a classic treatise on acupuncture and other Chinese medicine, written in 480-222 B.C.

Meridians

In acupuncture there are twelve meridians or pathways of energy—connecting points on the body and running up and down the body. In our embryonic development, all body organs send a nerve plexus to the skin. Hence, each organ has a number of corresponding points on the skin. An example of how we experience this is a condition of the heart known as angina pectoris. When the heart is experiencing difficulties one often feels pain radiating up the left arm into the pectoral muscle. This could represent a warning of a lack of coronary circulation and a pending heart attack.

By introducing one of the forms of stimulus (needles, electricity, laser, essential oils, heat, or pressure) in acupuncture the affected organ can be changed with regard to its function. We know as well that certain organs are closely related to other specific organs and they operate in unison. This is a fact that explains some of the connections of organs by meridians in acupuncture. This represents the process of "balance and harmony" within the body. If someone possesses a scar on the skin through a meridian it is possible to experience a disruption of the flow of energy to the corresponding organ.

Metal Fillings in Teeth

This also explains why I have seen disturbance in an organ when the meridian for that organ travels through a specific tooth that has a cavity filled with certain incompatible metals. There seems to be a relationship here that requires more research. In the meantime, caution should be taken in selecting the type of filling that goes into the tooth. Use composite materials or gold. Also, consider the removal of specific teeth when there is disease in the corresponding organ and the tooth contains metals that are incompatible with proper electrical conduction.

Use of Ears in Acupuncture

Taking acupuncture a step further, it was discovered by the Chinese and refined by a French physician, Dr. Paul Nogier, that all the meridians and organs have connections with the ear. Not only that, but the ear becomes a miniature map of the entire body — the ridge in the ear corresponding to the vertebrae, etc. — the entire body being molded in the ear; a sort of microcosm; or a "hologram", if you will. Hence, by treating a specific point on the ear the equivalent part of the body is affected. If pain exists in the back, when the specific point in the ear is treated, I have observed complete remission of the pain — sometimes within minutes.

Pain Relief

At times the effect is only temporary; sometimes it can be permanent. This brings to the forefront one of the most popular and useful functions of acupuncture — pain relief. In some cases where everything else has failed, I have seen complete relief of pain by using acupuncture. Its effects can be so profound that it is possible to perform surgery on a patient being treated with acupuncture. Visiting physicians have observed major surgery being performed in China with acupuncture the only anesthesia. It is certainly much safer than drugs, and in the United States a few anesthesiologists are using this technique.

The School of Medicine at the University of California at Los Angeles (UCLA) has implemented acupuncture as one of its modalities under the leadership of Dr. Richard Kroening, medical director of the Pain Management Clinic and assistant professor of anesthesiology. I had the privilege of training at the outpatient clinic of UCLA and was very impressed with the results of acupuncture in cases of acute or chronically resistant pain, particularly when all other therapies had failed.

Summary of Acupuncture

While many therapies have come and gone, acupuncture has certainly withstood the test of time (over 5,000 years), indicating its value.

I feel that in cases of persistent pain, acupuncture should be tried first, not only as a last resort as so often happens. It is certainly much safer than most drugs. For those persons who are squeamish about needles, even the tiniest ones, electrical acupuncture should be tried, as the skin is not invaded.

In summary, acupuncture represents a safe, effective way to treat health problems and certainly should be considered in many medical situations as a complementary therapy of great value.

✺ MANIPULATION OF THE BODY

Manipulation is the act of a therapist moving the muscles, skeletal system, tendons, ligaments, and viscera in order to achieve beneficial results for the patient. Medical doctors, osteopaths, chiropractors, myopractors, and massage therapists are practicing these techniques.

Spine and Lower Back Pain

What can manipulation do? Obviously, if the spine is out of alignment the pressure on nerves to organs and other parts of the body could cause severe pain and malfunction. This is particularly true when there already exists some type of pathology, such as a disc problem of the back, etc. Low back pain, which is very common, is particularly helped by adjustment and manipulation of the spine.

Ribs

Ribs may be displaced, which impairs smooth respiration and causes pain. Sometimes after rib manipulation breathing eases and the heart seems to operate better.

Short leg
Cases of one leg being shorter than the other are frequently caused by a displaced pelvis or rotated spine. Sometimes pelvis or spinal manipulation can correct this problem.

Scoliosis
Manipulation can also help scoliosis (curvature of the spine), particularly in people less than thirty years of age, when calcification of the spine normally begins. The consequences of calcification is a fixation of the spine.

Head Injury
The cranium or skull contains bones that move ever so subtly with respiration. This helps pump the cerebral spinal fluid through the spinal cord and around the brain. Through a head injury, the bones of the skull may be misaligned or fixed. In many patients they can be loosened if treated prior to the total calcification of the cranium.

Calcium is truly a destroyer, and calcification, which occurs throughout life, is said to be the results of the end process of all diseases or advanced aging. I have observed many symptoms, including headaches and dizziness from a head injury, resolved after one cranial manipulation. Unfortunately, there are few good cranial therapists in the United States.

Visceral Manipulation
Lastly, visceral manipulation, a rather new field, offers much help in conditions such as hiatus or hiatal hernia and an abnormally functioning ileocecal valve, the valve separating the small intestine from the large intestine.

Summary of Manipulation
If you have any muscle or joint strains, aches, and pains, then consider adding manipulation to your health program. You could be relieved of much pain and suffering.

✒ Safe, Effective Health and Healing

Ultimately we must look at the whole person—body, mind, and spirit—in order to achieve safe and effective health and healing. We must also include sciences such as homeopathy, aromatherapy, acupuncture, and manipulation to complement our health.

REFERENCES:

Barral, Jean-Pierre and Pierre Mercier. *Visceral Manipulation.* Seattle: Eastland Press, 1988.

CHAPTER 7

Aromatherapy

AROMATHERAPY IS AN ART and a science that has been practiced for several thousand years. Historical records reveal that the ancient Egyptians developed and promoted the use of oils for their citizenry.

In 1991 I toured the ancient temples and pyramids of Egypt. While exploring these magnificent structures and museums, I found evidence of a population with surprisingly advanced knowledge of medicine and healing and a deep understanding of the complexities of the human body. It may initially be surprising to learn that oils were used in sacred ceremonies as well as for healing the body of disease. Indeed, in the Egyptian culture ancient physicians were priests first.

There is abundant evidence of the frequent use of frankincense, myrrh, sandalwood, and rose oils in ancient Egypt. The discovery of these oils among other treasures of gold and silver within the sealed tombs is further indication of the value placed on them by this culture.

References in both the Old and New Testaments of the Bible include the application of frankincense, sandalwood, and patchouly to bless and purify the body. The Scripture also recommends hyssop, myrrh, and cinnamon for reversal of infectious diseases and protection against plagues.

❧ How Do Essential Oils Work?

As we learn more about vibratory rates of substances, we begin to understand why these oils can be used successfully in sacred ceremonies and in healing the body, as well as in many other applications. Applying an oil of a particular vibratory rate on an individual will raise the vibratory rate of a specific organ or the body upon which it is used. Diffusing an oil of a particular vibratory rate raises the level of oxygen and thus the energy within a room. Raising the vibration results in restoring health to the body, clarity to the mind, and attunement to the spirit. This occurs because the molecules that make up the structure of the oils vibrate at a specific frequency, or rate of movement. These frequencies are measured by using highly sensitive instruments. Each oil is unique and has its own specific frequency from 52 to 320 megahertz. Rose oil is the highest at 320 megahertz.

Today, with the appearance of new diseases caused by unknown microbes including viruses, bacteria, fungi and parasites, the use of these oils is appropriate and, possibly, critical to our health. This is particularly important since many of our antibiotics no longer have significant affect against these microbes. This problem is further complicated because many new, virulent strains of old diseases have evolved as a result of the misuse and/or overuse of antibiotics. In fact the Food and Drug Administration recently released a statement that their biggest concern in health care today is protecting citizens from many new and resistant diseases. Oils, used successfully in ancient times to combat the spread of disease, are successful agents today in combating the effects of even the newest pathogens.

This brings up yet another reason for using oils to maintain our health. Many of the ancient ailments thought to have disappeared, including the plague, have returned with a vengeance. Examples of oils that may protect us from such pathogens are clove, lemon, eucalyptus, and oregano.

Another reason to consider the essential oils is that they represent a natural modality of healing. Many synthetic drugs, including anti-inflammatory and other arthritis drugs, those for digestive ailments and gastritis, antihypertensives, diuretics, antiallergy, cholesterol-lowering agents, and so on, have potentially serious side effects. In fact

$77 billion is spent annually on drug-related complications. In addition, because of our toxic environment, our bodies have become so sensitive and overloaded that they are unable in some cases to properly break down and eliminate the chemical residue of these drugs from our bodies. We should be committed to looking for safe and natural alternatives for healing the body.

Since the United States has been behind the rest of the scientifically developed countries in regards to Aromatherapy, I traveled to Turkey in 1996. There I studied aromatherapy at the Ismir University. Turkey is wonderfully situated on the Mediterranean with diverse climate and topography of plains, sea coasts, and mountains. Toxic chemicals for the most part are not used on the land. In fact, McCormick, the company that markets spices, has a large processing operation is Ismir.

While there I learned of the proper application of the essential oils for many clinical conditions. I learned how the plants are grown, harvested, and distilled. This information is invaluable in my medical application of the essential oils.

Where do we get these oils? The essential oils come from plants. Any portion of the bush, flower, herb, or tree can be used as long as it produces an oil substance. The stem, flower, branches, leaves, or roots are also utilized, and oils may be derived from tree sap or bark.

After the oils are harvested, they are distilled using the specific temperature, pressure, and length of time suitable to each. Extracting the essential oils in this manner conserves their healing abilities.

The primary characteristics of these oils are as carriers of nutrients for the body and as sources of oxygen for the tissues and organs. This has tremendous value in stimulating our immune system. It is well known that human tissues require a substantial concentration of oxygen for their health. The oxygen and other nutrients are carried efficiently by the oils assuring good nutrition and, consequently, better health of the body tissues.

Oils play much the same role in plants that blood plays in the human body. As is true with humans, plants are also subjected to a variety of insects, fungi, bacteria, and viruses. Just as our blood stream carries nutrients throughout our body to keep us healthy, the oil or resin of the plants protects them and keeps them healthy.

✤ How Are Essential Oils Administered?

Oils may be administered in numerous ways. Inhalation is the process most used. As essential oils are inhaled, they make their way through the nasal passages by way of the nasal mucosa to the receptors of the brain or into the lungs where they are absorbed into the blood stream. Because the human body has between 10,000 to 100,000 more storage sites in the limbic system of smell than the senses of sight, touch, and taste combined, can there be any doubt that the oils may have a tremendously stimulating effect on the body functions?

This is why one of the most effective ways of delivering the oils for inhalation is through diffusion. A diffusor is a mechanical device that breaks up the oil into tiny particles and distributes them into the air. This is a valuable method for continuously receiving the benefits of the oils.

Oils may also be applied directly to the skin over an injured area requiring special support. This is indicated whether the problem is painful joints, ligaments, or bones, or specific organs or tissues of the body requiring added assistance. This includes the lymphatic, circulatory, digestive, and urinary or water elimination systems, as well as the nervous and respiratory systems.

Localized injuries of the skin, such as abrasions, lacerations, burns, scars, or infections respond well to the direct application of oils such as lavender, chamomile, or melrose. All of these problems will benefit from direct application or diffusion of essential oils.

You may potentiate the healing effect by layering one oil over another, which may bring the desired result more quickly. A number of the stronger oils should be diluted with a carrier oil such as cold-pressed olive oil, or almond oil. Oils such as frankincense or lavender may be applied by themselves. Oils such as cinnamon, clove, lemon, and eucalyptus may be blended together to amplify their affects and hence achieve healing more completely.

Oils may also be placed on the skin over specific energy points. Meridians or acupuncture lines have been known for thousands of years by the Chinese. The energy running through these lines, as they are referred to here, end in various places on the body. One of the major ending points of the meridians are the soles of the feet. Each organ or body structure is identified on the body map illustrated on the soles of the feet. They are referred to as vitaflex points.

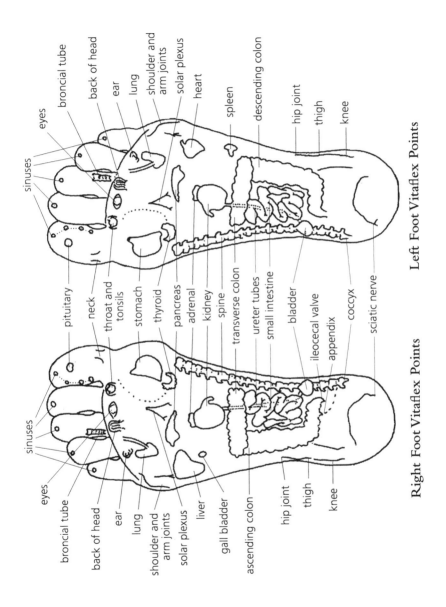

Left Foot Vitaflex Points

Right Foot Vitaflex Points

Application of oils or physical stimulation with needles or low voltage electricity on these vitaflex points can produce changes in the corresponding organ.

Another application of the oils is by a rectal implant. This is accomplished by inserting the oils rectally with a soft rubber syringe bulb. A rectal implant would be of value in the case of an enlarged or congested prostate gland, which is located near the rectum. In this case, a combination of frankincense, myrrh, and sage oils at a proportion of 10, 5, and 3 drops with one teaspoon of carrier oil would be recommended. This may be done at bedtime for 10 days, then therapy is suspended for 4 days, then this cycle is repeated once again for greater affect.

In Europe the essential oil Vitex, which is derived from the chase tree is used to treat Parkinsonism. According to the French physician Dr. Jean Claude LaPraz, he has observed an 89 percent success rate in reversing the symptoms of this dreaded disease. He recommended inhaling Vitex and applying it to the spine and soles of the feet.

Melissa essential oil has been found effective in treating viruses. It is particularly helpful in counteracting Herpes Simplex, which some of us know as cold sores the form around the lips, and Herpes Genitalis, in which blisters are found around the genitals.

Melissa has also been shown to improve the behavior of hyperactive children. Today 3 to 5 percent of the students in our school system take a drug called Ritalin to treat this condition. Perhaps we should investigate the benefits of Melissa as a natural therapeutic adjunct.

❀ The Essential Oils and their Actions

In the following chart I have listed some of the most important oils and oil blends and how they may help support our bodies with their specific actions. These are just a few of the oils that may help support the system when used used in these conditions.

These oils may be placed on location (at the site of the problem), placed on the vitaflex points on the soles of the feet, or inhaled through diffusion. I recommend that all three applications be used when the maximum benefits are desired.

Condition	Effective Oils or Blends	Application
Attention Deficit Disorder (ADD)	Lavender	bottom of feet, massage, diffuse
Allergies	Lavender and Chamomile, Eucalyptus	sinus area, bottom of feet, diffuse
Antibiotic	Bergamot, Roman Chomille, Clove, Hyssop, Oregano, Myrtle, Cinnamon, Ravensara, Melaleuca	on location, liver, on bottom of feet
Antihistamine	Lavender and Roman Chomille	vitaflex points, sinuses, diffuse
Arterial vasal dilation and hypertension	Helichrysum, Ylang ylang and Marjoram	vitaflex points, heart, back, diffuse
Arthritis	Birch, Helichrysum	on location, vitaflex points
Asthma	Ravensara, Lavender, Frankincense	lungs, throat, on pillow, diffuse
Back, alignment and pain	Basil, Birch, Cypress, and Raindrop Therapy (see Glossary)	on location, vitaflex points
Bites, insect	Cinnamon, Peppermint	on location
Bronchitis	Ylang ylang, Patchouly	lungs, diffuse
Burns	Lavender	on location
Candida	Mountain Savory, Melaleuca	chest, lungs, bottom of feet
Digestive difficulties	Peppermint, Tarragon, Juniper, Ansum, Fennel	stomach, abdomen, few drops in food
Edema	Tangerine, Cypress, Juniper	inner legs ankles to knee (lower extremities), bottom of feet
Energy	Lemon	shoulders, solar plexus, bottom of feet, diffuse
Hair, to stimulate growth	Cypress, Lemon, Ylang ylang	massage on scalp, use in shampoo
Headaches	Peppermint, Helichrysum	on location, bottom of feet, diffuse

Condition	Effective Oils or Blends	Application
Hearing, to improve	Helichrysum and Juniper	bottom of feet, two small toes, small fingers, ear canal, mastoid*
Hyperactivity	Lavender	bottom of feet, thymus, diffuse
Immune System, to boost	Frankincense, Oregano	bottom of feet, along spine, diffuse under arms,
Insomnia	Lavender	bottom of feet, temples, diffuse
Ligaments, sore	Lemongrass	on location
Lymphatic, to improve	Lemon	vitaflex points, upper spine, thymus
Memory, to improve	Rose, Basil	on temples, diffuse
Mental fatigue	Basil	temples, back of neck, diffuse
Muscle aches	Birch	on location, bottom of feet
Sinusitis	Myrtle, Eucalyptus	sinus, temples, chest, neck, back, vitaflex point, sinuses
Stretch marks	Lavender, Myrrh	on location
Sunburn	Melaleuca, Lavender	on location
Viruses	Oregano, Thyme	along spine, bottom of feet,
Vision, to improve	Lemongrass, Cypress, Eucalyptus,	eyebrows (not in eyes) big toes, thumbs, diffuse, thymus

*Note: Never pour hot oil into the ear.

❦ EMOTIONS

Aromatherapy literally means to therapeutically treat the individual by inhaling the oils. The olfactory bulb is responsible for detection of odors. The mucous membranes are located inside the passageway of the nose and make a connection to the olfactory nerves. The very small airborne oil droplets stimulate the nerve receptors of the olfactory bulb and transmit both the micro-fine oil particles and the messages from the frequency of the oils to the brain. This ends in the mid-brain portion called the limbic system. This is the portion of the brain responsible for the sense of smell. The emotional part of the limbic system of the brain is called the amygdala.

In 1989 Dr. Ledoux of New York Medical University made a discovery that significantly determines how we look at emotions. He discovered that emotions are connected and perhaps stored in the amygdala. Further investigation revealed that the emotional release of a trauma situation may be simplified by odors, which also act upon this part of the brain. How many times have specific smells reminded us of events? The smell of foods baking can cause us to recall a pleasant situation such as a visit with our family during the holidays. This may be equally applied to negative situations.

It has been my experience in medicine that the memory of emotional trauma should be released for one to heal and get on with one's life. If these emotional traumas are retained in our consciousness they may interfere with our health, particularly when they are perceived as unpleasant, life-threatening, or negative situations. It is the opinion of some psychologists that the most detrimental action is to suppress these emotions. I have observed that, by using specific oils, patients may recall and deal with certain emotionally charged events so the negative energy to ultimately be released.

Listed below are some of the major emotions and several of the most effective oils that I have used to balance them.

Emotion	Effective Oils	Application
Abundance	Angelica, Spruce, Myrrh, Patchouly, Rose, Frankincense	heart, solar plexus, diffuse
Abuse	Frankincense, Geranium, Lavender, Rose, Citrus	soles of feet, throat, forehead, diffuse
Anger	Ylang ylang, Lavender, Sandalwood	soles of feet, liver, throat shoulders, forehead, diffuse

Emotion	Effective Oils	Application
Apathy	Rose, Ylang ylang, Citrus, Angelica, Frankincense, Hyssop, Spruce, Lavender, Sandalwood, Melissa	heart, soles of feet, kidneys, forehead, diffuse
Bitterness	Roman Chamomile, Sandalwood, Lavender, Ylang ylang	heart, soles of feet
Compassion	Helichrysum	heart, diffuse
Depression	Frankincense, Rose, Juniper, Melissa	forehead, top of head, diffuse
Fear	Angelica, Rose, Melissa, Juniper, Ylang ylang, Citrus, Bergamot, Neroli	kidneys, abdomen, liver, soles of feet, heart
Forgiveness	Frankincense, Ylang ylang, Cardamon, Rosemary, Peppermint, Rose, Melissa, Helichrysum, Spruce	temples, heart, soles of feet, back of neck, diffuse
Grief, sorrow	Citrus, Ylang ylang, Rose, Frankincense, Melissa, Helichrysum, Bergamot, Rosewood	heart, chest, abdomen, diffuse
Guilt	Rosewood, Frankincense, Ylang ylang, Spruce, Neroli, Rose, Melissa	heart, thymus, solar plexus, kidneys, liver, soles of feet, diffuse
Habits, to break	Lavender	abdomen, heart, diffuse
Irritability	Rose, Rosewood, Frankincense, Spruce, Ylang ylang, Juniper, Angelica, Neroli, Tanactum, Melissa, Helichrysum	abdomen, shoulders, top of head, back of neck, diffuse
Joy	Rose, Citrus, Ylang ylang	heart, diffuse
Obsessiveness Rosewood,	Rose, Sandalwood, solar plexus, diffus Tanactum, Frankincense	kidneys, soles of feet,
Panic	Harmony, Angelica, Hyssop, Rosewood, Tanactum, Frankincense, Spruce, Lavender, Geranium	heart, kidneys, soles of feet, under nose, diffuse

Emotion	Effective Oils	Application
Procrastination	Neroli, Sandalwood, Tanactum, Rosewood, Ylang ylang, Spruce	bottom of feet, thymus, diffuse
Protection	Angelica, Frankincense, Sandalwood, Rose	shoulders, abdomen, soles of feet, diffuse
Relaxation	Clary Sage, Palmarose, Geranium, Chamomile, Rose, Citrus, Ylang ylang, Tanactum	soles of feet, diffuse
Resentment	Hyssop, Spruce, Lavender, Rosewood, Acceptance, Ylang ylang, Citrus, Frankincense	heart, forehead, liver, abdomen, diffuse
Sadness	Orange, Sandalwood, Rose, Citrus, Ylang ylang, Juniper, Bergamot, Frankincense	heart, soles of feet, forehead, thorax
Self esteem, to improve	Rose, Citrus, Ylang ylang	soles of feet, wrists, diffuse
Self love	Rose, Bergamot, Citrus, Ylang ylang, Juniper, Frankincense, Sandalwood,	heart, top of head, diffuse
Spiritual attunement	Frankincense, Sandalwood, Juniper, Rose	center of forehead, top of head, temples, neck, diffuse
Stress	Basil, Bergamot, Geranium, Grapefruit, Lavender	soles of feet, temples, diffuse
Tension	Citrus, Ylang ylang, Tanactum, Patchouly, Hyssop, Spruce, Lavender	heart, diffuse
Trauma, mental, to release	Rose, Juniper, Ylang ylang, Citrus, Bergamot, Sandalwood, Lavender, Frankincense	soles of feet, heart, diffuse
Trauma, emotional, to release	Geranium, added to above	soles of feet, diffuse

Emotion	Effective Oils	Application
Well-being	Lemon, Citrus, Angelica, Ylang ylang, Lavender, Sandalwood, Geranium, Hyssop, Spruce, Melissa, Juniper	soles of feet, temples, heart

❧ OTHER POSITIVE EFFECTS OF THE ESSENTIAL OILS

Another very important attribute of the oils is their ability to enhance oral nutrients. As I stated earlier the oils contain oxygen and when oxygen is delivered to the tissues of the body, this improves the actions of the nutrients. In fact, many nutrients require oxygen to fulfill their functions.

The oils also have the ability to act as antioxidants, hence they assist in removal of potentially pathological chemicals that are created during cellular and tissue metabolism. These so-called free radicals also occur as the result of the body's effort to remove xenobiotics or abnormal chemicals, heavy metals, and other noxious substances.

It is known that free radical damage poses an on-going threat to health because of damage both to the cell wall due to the presence of these and other toxins, and of large numbers of pathological microbes and miscellaneous debris in the tissues surrounding the cells. The essential oils, however, act to dissipate these barriers by destroying those tiny microbes and oxidizing the debris.

When the oils are added to foods, the absorption, assimilation, and utilization of the nutrients greatly improves and consequently repairs much of the free radical damage. In addition, the oils are able to better penetrate the walls of the cells and hence carry the nutrients into the cells. This includes vitamins, minerals, enzymes, fats, proteins, and carbohydrates. All of these products are essential for the health of the cells and their longevity.

🌿 THE QUALITY OF ESSENTIAL OILS

It is imperative that all the products I use to treat my patients be of the highest possible quality and purity. As a physician, I feel that it is mandatory that I personally investigate and ultimately feel confident that the products I use and recommend unequivocally meet my high standards. Furthermore, as a member of the American Medical Association, I abide by their bylaws and code of ethics, which prohibits the physician's recommendation of products in which he or she has a financial interest. An exception to this rule is recognized when the products recommended are of such high quality and uniqueness that they are generally unavailable from any other source.

Such is the case with the products used in aromatherapy. In my opinion, no one in the United States has done more to bring out the wonderful healing qualities of oils than Gary Young, owner of Young Living Essential Oils. I have personally walked in the fields that produce the plants that afford these excellent oils, I have attended their careful harvest and participated in the distillation of their oils. My judgement that these oils are the best available comes from my experience with this family farm and my early studies at the University of Illinois in the school of chemical engineering. I am continually impressed with the purity of these essential oils and the quality control of their processing. And after years of utilizing these oils in my clinic, I have found them to be highly effective therapeutically.

Young was a naturopathic physician who had his own clinic in Chula Vista, Calif. He tried diligently to find new ways to reverse the ailments of many chronically ill individuals who had failed to get relief from other physicians or methodologies. After his own personal health crises, he began to explore alternative methods that were natural and harmonious with the body. In 1983, he studied and initiated research on tee tree oil, commonly called melaleuca. He incorporated this oil into his practice. In order to further study the benefits of essential oils, he attended seminars in Switzerland and in other parts of Europe. There he learned of the many benefits of these and other oils from medical doctors who had used essential oils for many years. They had combined the research and the historical data on the value of the oils from both present medical research and research of ancient records.

When looking for similar research done in the United States, Gary found there was essentially no one in this country who possessed adequate knowledge of the oils, especially with respect to their healing qualities. Secondly, he found that when he used a poor quality oil, grade 4 or 5 oil as rated by the experts who have knowledge of the oils, he had little or no results in healing applications. When he used first or second quality oil, he found that his results were substantially higher.

Many of the oils that were available in the eighties were not of first quality, as is the case today. It is much cheaper to distill oils if it is not necessary to take care during the distillation process. However, the oils produced are primarily of perfume grade, satisfactory if you are using oils simply for cosmetic purposes. However, for healing to occur it is necessary to have a first or second grade oil.

For example, frankincense resin is sold in Somalia at costs between $30,000 to 35,000 a pound. However, frankincense sold for $25 an ounce, for example, has been distilled with alcohol and is much less affective in healing than an oil that is distilled at a proper temperature, pressure, and time. When these oils are cut synthetically, which means chemically produced in a laboratory and therefore adulterated, it not only reduces the healing ability, but produces rashes, a burning sensation, and other skin irritations when applied. You will find many so-called aromatherapists that state that all oils must be diluted before being applied to the skin, though this is simply because they are using lower quality oils.

Unfortunately, most people do not have the knowledge to distinguish good quality oils from poor quality oils, and many of the oils are mislabeled. Ten years ago there were 26 to 30 distilling sources in Europe. Today no more than two or three are still in operation, for the cost of producing a high-quality oil has sky rocketed. At the same time, there is a great deal of cheap and diluted oil coming from countries such as China and India. These oils are not only less expensive, but the quality of the oils is less than we would desire to use therapeutically.

CHAPTER 8

The Immune System—
Under Attack and Defending

OUR WORLD PRESENTS a hostile environment that increasingly stresses and weakens our immune system, our primary line of defense against disease. We must be cognizant of the dangers confronting us. In the following pages you will learn how you may nourish and strengthen your immune system, as well as how you may reverse acute and chronic debilitating diseases. The five-step program I have developed will assist you in achieving good health.

⚕ INFECTIOUS DISEASES

Today, a large number of environmental stresses are attacking our body's immune system. Because of these stresses and the sudden emergence of new and highly virulent infectious diseases, our health is being challenged severely.

A report was recently released by Vice President Al Gore. It stated in part:

> An area in which tremendous strides have been made is the fight against infectious disease. Progress has been so great that three decades ago some predicted that we would soon see the end of infectious dis-

ease epidemics. However, infectious diseases are re-emerging around the globe, including in the United States. In the past decade, we have seen HIV/AIDS explode into a global pandemic. Other diseases thought to be under control are re-emerging worldwide, such as tuberculosis, cholera, and pneumonia. The factors that contribute to the resurgence of these diseases — the evolution of drug-resistant microbes, population movement, changes in ecology and climate — show no sign of abatement.

New viruses are attacking us constantly. Every year millions of people contract the flu, and many die as a consequence of its complications. One reason the flu is difficult to prevent and cure is that the virus mutates radically every year, forming new strains. For instance, the Marburg virus outbreak, which attacked the nervous system and stomach, caused infected victims to suffer a painful death by internal bleeding.

Recently, the news media reported an infection similar to the Marburg virus, the deadly Ebola viral infection that broke out in Zaire, Africa. Authorities from the World Health Organization rushed to Zaire in an effort to contain the deadly virus and stop it from spreading to other countries. Why? Because each person infected has a 90 percent chance of becoming a fatality statistic.

With airline travel readily available to the mass population from the Amazon to Africa, someone who contracted a virus in a foreign nation could be in New York City the same day they became infected. In addition, with the continuous recycling of the oxygen on airplanes, every passenger and crew member could contract the disease or become a carrier. With many passengers transferring to other planes to reach their final destination, the potential for starting a widespread epidemic not only exists, but seems inevitable.

However, it is not only these new viruses about which we should be concerned. In recent years old diseases considered extinct are again rearing their ugly heads and threatening to cause new epidemics. These include diphtheria, cholera, anthrax, tuberculosis, and "the plague." Both in medieval Europe and as late as the early 1900s, we were led to believe that these germs were a problem only because of inadequate sanitation and poor personal hygiene. Even though both of these contributed to the spread of disease, it has been discovered that they were not the exclusive cause of the problem. Of course, antibiotics had not yet been discovered to aid in the control of such diseases.

With the advance of antibiotics, many of these diseases were cured, and some all but obliterated. However, because of the widespread and inexcusable overuse of antibiotics, many infectious organisms have developed resistant strains. Tuberculosis is a good example of an organism that has created a new, highly resistant strain that has baffled doctors and other scientists during the last 15 years.

Even our water supplies, upon which we are so dependent because they are critical to our health and well-being, are becoming contaminated in some of America's largest cities. A serious outbreak of gastroenteritis occurred after the intestinal parasite Cryptosporidium parvum was found in the municipal drinking water of one city in 1993. Hundreds of people sought treatment at hospital emergency rooms, and many died because of compromised immune systems. Now, we are finding these same parasites in the drinking water of other large American cities, including New York and Phoenix.

Also, we just now are learning that the common gastric and duodenal ulcer is not caused merely by improper lifestyle, as previously thought. Actually, it was found that as high as 92 percent of duodenal ulcers are caused primarily by an infectious bacteria called *Heliobacter pylori*. This is a corkscrew-shaped bacteria that invades the gastrointestinal mucosa and secretes urease that, in turn, produces ammonia. This protects the bacteria against the effects of hydrochloric acid, which is secreted by the stomach to digest food. By neutralizing this acid, the bacteria is able to survive. Of course, this disrupts our digestion process.

One illness that exemplifies the complete failure of the immune system is AIDS.

The HIV virus invades the immune system and suppresses and cripples its function, limiting the body's ability to fight off infections. As we know, this usually ends in death. Without a cure, this disease is infecting more and more of the population, and the fact that it is spreading rapidly into all areas of every population is well publicized.

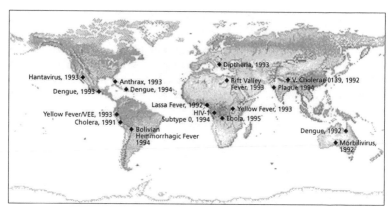

Viruses Around the World in Recent Years

🌿 Environmental Toxins

Inorganic toxins are another major cause of a depressed immune system. You frequently hear of toxins in our environment (air, soil, and food pollution) and the harm that they can do. Much is written about them and their effects, but most of us believe they can't really affect us all that seriously. However, we only have to look at what has happened to our major cities over the last several years. A dirty haze settles over them, and the Department of Environmental Quality has determined that air quality has reached unhealthful proportions in many cities. The reason cited is a major warm air/cold air inversion, trapping the pollution produced by wood-burning stoves and fireplaces, aerosol sprays, and thousands of cars. The increase in traffic is caused, of course, by the tremendous population growth in most of our major cities.

This problem is expected to continue, but the question is, "What are the physical consequences of air pollution?" Some people experience burning, itching, and infected eyes, sore throats, and bronchial coughs, which could lead to serious respiratory infections, as well as an increase in asthma, bronchitis, and pneumonia conditions.

Then there is the petro-chemical exposure in our environment; the amount of pesticides, herbicides, and other chemicals applied to our crops and landscaping is very high. The Environmental Protection Agency estimates that two pounds per acre of these products are added to our food crops yearly, five pounds to our neatly groomed lawns, and 15 to 40 pounds per acre of chemicals are applied to our golf courses. According to the National Institute of Health, grounds keepers and managers of country clubs suffer three times the incidence of lymphoma as the general population. Persons living on golf courses also have an increased risk of cancer and other diseases. We also may see serious neurological effects from these petrochemical toxins. These may include fever, nausea, weakness, tremors, flushing of the skin, dullness of concentration and thought, pounding heart, and numbness in the hands and feet.

Many of us also have been exposed to large amounts of heavy metals, such as mercury, lead, aluminum, and cadmium, all of which interfere with the health of our immune systems. Heavy metals are derived from amalgam fillings in our teeth or from the consumption of seafood, which is also high in mercury. In the case of lead, it is found in paints and was found in gasoline. Lead may damage the mitochondria that act as power plants for our muscles. This causes severe physical weakness and pain. Aluminum is found in underarm deodorants and aluminum cookware. Our society has extracted these toxic metals from below the earth's surface and spread them around on the surface of our planet and in our environment.

❦ The Immune System

We must consider the risks involved in drinking water and eating food. Many chemicals are found in these necessary and nourishing products. Our protection and defense against these diseases and toxins is the immune system. How does it work?

The term "immune" comes from the Latin word "immunist," which means "exempt from, resistant to, or protected from disease, infectious organisms, poisons, allergens, and other agents." Our bodies tend to defend themselves against any substance or particle that is foreign to them.

In response to stressors (anything causing stress), both physical (chemicals, bacteria, viruses, foods, pollens, or mold) and psychological, our brains release various substances that assist in the protection of the body.

Allergens are any environmental material. They can be inhalants (pollens, molds, animal dander, and insect parts), ingestants (foods and drugs), or contactants (hair dyes, cosmetics, and metals). We have two types of cells that generally react with allergens. These are "T" cells and "B" cells, each a type of antibody. Antibodies are proteins that protect the body by neutralizing the attacking substance (allergen). When the T cell is the mediator (arbitrator or go-between), we experience a dermal or skin reaction that is an inflammation caused by direct contact. We also can find this type of reaction with an inflammation of the lungs leading to pneumonitis secondary to hypersensitivity to an allergen.

The immune system is stimulated by way of the thymus gland and the bursal equivalents. Bursa equivalent is tissue similar to bursa. One line of defense is the B cells. The B cells derived from bursa of the body work with some lymphocytes and act as antigen receptors. The hormonal system contains the B cells. The B cells form the proteins. One of these proteins is IgE and it functions with antibody reaction to counteract an allergic substance or allergen. Products formed by these organs function to counteract the effects of the stressors.

Another important location for the immune system is the Peyer's Patches. These are groups of lymph nodules found mainly in the lower part of the small intestine. They lie in the three main regions of the lining of the intestine, the submucosa, mucosa, and mucosal villi. The villi are that part of the region that has the first contact with food and other products, hence intestinal absorption begins here. These patches are composed of lymphatic complexes and nodules. They grow in size and increase in function from birth until the age of ten years, then decrease with age. They include both thymus and bursa-derived cells and hence effect both IgM and IgG portions of the immune system. When babies and many young children pick up objects, the first place they go is into the mouth. This system is so important. We need this protection.

The IgM is made up of B cells and its action predominates in the early immune responses. The IgA is present in blood, saliva, colostrum, tears, and secretions of the bronchi as well as the gastrointestinal tract. It primarily defends the individual against viral and bacterial infections at the mucosal level of the system.

This plays a major role in our immune system because much of our defense system must interact with the products we ingest. How many times have we unknowingly consumed food or water that is contaminated with bacteria, viruses, fungi, parasites, and chemical toxins? This is a very important defense system for our bodies and, according to some scientific evidence, may represent 40 percent of our total immune system. Since it degenerates with age we may be more susceptible to these toxins and microbes in later life.

The bowels should be balanced with a normal helpful flora made up of bacteria. It should generally be free from fungi and pathological or harmful bacteria. Once the flora is normal an oral intake of homeopathic Peyer's Patches may reestablish the normal activity of this important portion of the immune system.

※ AUTOIMMUNITY

Autoimmune diseases cannot be explained by a solitary cause or mechanism. Small amounts of auto-antibodies normally are produced and may have physiological roles in cellular interactions. The major theories regarding the development of autoimmune diseases are (1) release of normal sequestered antigens (a portion of a virus, bacteria, etc.), (2) the presence of abnormal clones, (3) shared antigens between the host and microorganisms, and (4) defects in helper or suppressor cell functions.

Genetic susceptibility is also a likely determinant of autoimmune disease. In nearly all autoimmune diseases, multiple mechanisms of autoimmunity are operative, and the exact causes are unknown.

※ HUMORAL ANTIBODY-MEDIATED AUTOIMMUNITY

The existence of antireceptor (something that blocks messages to the body's organs) antibodies that compete with or mimic various physiologic antagonists for cellular receptors is a specific autoimmune mechanism in several diseases. In Graves' disease, a thyroid condition, antibodies are present that compete with thyroid cells and stimulate thyroid hormone production. In rare instances of type I diabetes mellitus, anti-insulin receptor antibodies cause insulin resistance in distant tissues.

❧ IMMUNE COMPLEX DISEASE

With this group of diseases (systemic lupus erythematosus, rheumatoid arthritis, some drug-induced hemolytic anemia, and thrombocytopenia), autologous or similar body tissues are injured as "innocent bystanders."

❧ SUPPORT AND REPAIR OF OUR IMMUNE SYSTEM

What must we do to support and repair our frequently dysfunctional immune system to protect ourselves against an onslaught of infectious diseases and environmental toxins? I have developed a five step program that, if followed, will enable patients to reverse their dysfunctional immune system and illnesses and create health and high-level wellness. I call this program the "5 R's":

1. Remove
2. Replace
3. Repair
4. Rejuvenate
5. Revitalize

Step One — Remove
In this step, "remove" also includes "avoid." Attempt to avoid toxins by staying indoors on high-pollution days. Avoid using chemicals and petro-chemically based sprays in and around your house. Bathe immediately after playing golf and wash your clothes. To neutralize your food, soak and wash your fruit and vegetables thoroughly, using a few drops of household bleach in a quart of water. Eliminate dyes and chemicals from your diet; read food labels. Drink only pure bottled water or, better yet, distilled and filtered water.

Remove the offending factors. If these factors are heavy metals, such as lead, cadmium, mercury, aluminum, or arsenic, chelate them out of the body. This is done by introducing a "chelating agent" into the system, which literally grabs the offending material and holds it in solution until the kidneys can flush it out. EDTA (Ethylene Diamine Tetra acetic Acid) is a very fine chelating agent when injected intravenously. EDTA is a protein that binds with all heavy metals and eliminates them safely, excreting them through the kidneys. An additional benefit is EDTA's ability to find and remove unwanted calcium that often clogs our arteries and impairs our circulation. Opening these arteries also improves the nutrition of body tissues.

DMPS (Dimercapto Propane Sulfonate) is also a powerful chelating agent and has a. high affinity for the metal mercury. However, if the factors are primarily pesticides and other chemicals, use this with dry sauna treatments. The largest area of excretion of the body is the skin. Heat causes elimination of toxins through perspiration. These toxins are trapped in the fatty tissue of the body and one of the easiest and quickest ways to remove them is by saunas.

If your stomach and bowels are infected with the bacteria *Heliobacter pylori* and other parasites such as protozoa and worms, or yeasts and other fungi, then these must be eliminated. If the body is already immune-compromised, then safe and natural products must be used instead of damaging antibiotics. I devised such a program using bentonite with colloidal silver that is mild and inoffensive to the body, but is devastating to many parasites and bacteria, including *Heliobacter pylori*.

Sometimes we are allergic to certain foods. These foods may cause injury to the intestinal mucosa. The result could be damage to the integrity of the filtering system of the mucosa, causing enlargement of these natural openings and admitting large molecular toxins and undigested food. The human digestive system often interprets these large molecules as foreign bodies and reacts in an allergic manner to the food particles. Therefore, once they are identified, these foods must be eliminated from the diet until the immune system is repaired and strengthened.

We also should include in our diet a mixed bran roughage consisting of various grains. These foods mechanically "brush" the intestinal tract, cleansing it of unwanted debris.

I also recommend a highly nutritional three or five-day fast, under a doctor's care. The fast recommended is the Master Cleanse, using

8–12 glasses per day of a mixture of:
    2 tbsp. grade "C" maple syrup
    2 tbsp. freshly squeezed lemon or lime juice
    ⅛ tsp. cayenne pepper
    8 oz. distilled water

Step Two — Replace

The second step is to replace the products that may be diminished or missing in our gastrointestinal system. One must reinoculate the intestines. Studies show that in sickness, the bowels usually contain an improper balance of bacterial growth. Over 300 species of beneficial bacteria grow symbiotically (working together in harmony) in our intestinal tract.

Another very important process in the "replacing" step is to assure that you have adequate enzymes for food digestion and assimilation of the nutrients. The major enzymes are pancreatin, lipase, trypsin, and hydrochloric acid, though this is only a partial list of enzymes. It should be understood that many of the B vitamins are converted by these enzymes, along with the normal intestinal bacteria, into a usable form of vitamin B, which is so necessary for your body's proper metabolism, growth, and energy.

It is very important to assure that your body has adequate glutathione, a tripeptide that functions in the liver. Glutathione detoxifies and neutralizes chemical products that cause damage to the body. These are called xenobiotics, e.g. any foreign products that are chemically unfriendly to the body. Assuring adequate glutathione protects the body against these products and reverse the aging process.

Step Three — Repair

Now that the digestive and detoxification systems are in place, we must repair the immune system and eliminate the end products of metabolism (waste and debris). We can initiate this process by using antioxidants and free radical scavengers. These are vitamins A, C, and E, selenium (a trace mineral), and pycnogenol. The latter is known as a powerful product derived from either grape seed extract or the bark of a pine tree that grows in northern France. These products not only should be taken as a function of this "repair" process, but also as elements of a maintenance program to protect the body.

The nutrients that are the building blocks of the body participate in this rebuilding process. These nutrients include minerals, both macro- and micro-, basically encompassing all of the minerals. This, of course, excludes the heavy metals such as lead, cadmium, aluminum, and mercury that may interfere with, rather than support, metabolism of the structures.

Another class of necessary building blocks is the amino acids. These basic proteins are the essential foundation of body tissue, and many of these biochemical products are found in our systems. Most of the amino acids must be taken orally.

Step Four— Rejuvenate
This implies not only the rejuvenation and regeneration of tissues, but organs as well. One recent finding is that the organs are unable to make adequate the hormones so necessary for body functions to occur properly when we are under duress.

DHEA (dehydroepiandrosterone) is a significant representation of this. It has been called the "mother hormone" because it is the raw material from which our bodies make estrogen, testosterone, progesterone, and corticosterone. The DHEA level in the blood reaches its peak at 20 years of age and declines with aging. Studies show that some people have premature low levels of DHEA. These same people often experience loss of energy, declining function, and accelerated aging, as well as an increase in degenerative diseases. Conversely, studies show that having acceptable levels of DHEA can prevent or reverse many diseases.

Dr. Elizabeth Barrett-Connor, M.D., from the University of California School of Medicine in San Diego, found a "48 percent reduction in cardiovascular disease and a 36 percent reduction in mortality from any cause" when DHEA levels were increased to the therapeutic levels. According to Dr. Barrett-Connor, DHEA protects the body by inhibiting the enzyme (glucose-6 phosphate dehydrogenase) that normally accelerates the production of both damaging fatty acids and cholesterol.

Other studies reveal that with DHEA significant diseases, such as cancer, obesity, depression, high blood pressure, diabetes, arthritis, senility, and Alzheimer's disease, can either be improved or reversed. There are also studies indicating that DHEA may be significant in improving memory and stimulating the immune system. Other studies taken during weight-loss programs have suggested that DHEA may be of significance in the fat-burning process, possibly by replacing fat with muscle tissue.

The best news is that when taken orally in prescribed doses, DHEA causes no toxicity. Because DHEA is an unpatentable drug, no major pharmaceutical company is interested in informing us of its value and/or marketing it. It is a prescription drug, and a recent report from the FDA claims that it will become a controlled substance. This means it must be used under the direction of a licensed M.D. and purchased from a registered pharmacist.

I recommend that the DHEA blood level be evaluated prior to its administration to determine whether or not there is, indeed, a significant decline of your DHEA level. A lack of DHEA could be the cause of your illness, and this is a dramatic and safe therapy available to you.

Second, the regeneration step should include purified tissue extracts such as liver, adrenal, and thyroid. These "extract" doses should be low, or even homeopathic. The latter is defined as a product diluted many times, sometimes resulting in only the molecular energy of the original product existing in distilled water. In either case, the benefit of the tissue extracts are found in their ability to restore and rebuild the organs that are damaged and, hence, not functioning properly. Particularly in the instance of homeopathic remedies, their function may be to act as a "blueprint material"—one that sends a message to the body as to how to rebuild the tissues and organs. In some cases, it furnishes raw material for this function as well.

When there has been severe damage, I use live-cell therapy. This involves administering the thymus gland cells of an unborn sheep or cow. The effect of this therapy is similar to doing an organ transplant, except that it is noninvasive, safer, and simpler. This rebuilds our own thymus gland, enabling it to function at a beneficial level, instead of its frequently dysfunctional level.

We also can restore greatly the mitochondria of a muscle cell that has been damaged by heavy metals and other xenobiotics, particularly petro-chemicals. This damage could lead to severe muscle fatigue and diseases such as fibromyalgia. Adding high doses of the natural product Coenzyme Q10 stimulates the activity of the muscles, assisting them to function normally. This also holds true for the heart muscle, stimulating it after it has become damaged, flabby, or poorly functioning. Hence, Coenzyme Q10 may improve the heart's function and may reverse serious debilitating heart disease.

There is a very important therapy to consider in rejuvenation. It involves an intravenous injection of ortho-molecular nutrients, specifically high doses of vitamin C (in the range of 100,000 - 450,000 mg.). This is 100 percent absorbed, unlike oral doses. It will generate rapid healing and destroy infections from viruses, bacteria, and fungi. The high dose of vitamin C apparently jump-starts the body and kicks the immune system into high gear. In addition to vitamin C, essential minerals and vitamin B are included and administered simultaneously. Generally, this therapy is given for five consecutive days. In many cases, the results are phenomenal.

Step Five — Revitalize

The fifth and last step of this program is to revitalize the body. First of all, we should have a good diet consisting of many vegetables, whole grains, some whole fruit, and protein from beans and brown rice. If you are not a vegetarian, protein also may come from fish and turkey. Less than 15 percent of the caloric intake of the diet should come from polyunsaturated fats that are not excessively heated. We should reduce or eliminate red meats, fried foods, salt, sugar, and refined and overprocessed foods. It is very important to drink eight or more glasses of pure water daily.

Exercise is very important. After approval is obtained from your physician, exercise for at least 20 minutes, four times a week. These exercise periods should be of a strenuous enough nature for you to perspire.

Essential oils are a very significant way to revitalize your body and elevate its function to an improved level. Now that we have everything operating properly, let's take it to high gear; the pure oils can take us there. Oils are one of the earliest forms of medicine. They were used in Egypt 4,000 years ago by the priest-physicians. Today, there is no other medicine with such a high frequency as the oils. Frequency is the energetic movement that a substance reflects as it vibrates.

We are in the age of energy medicine, and the body normally functions between a range of 50-75 megahertz, according to researcher Dr. Gary Young. Disease has frequency of 58 megahertz down (cancer 42 megahertz), which is one measurement of energy. To combat disease, we use various products. Drugs have a frequency of 0-10 megahertz. Herbs have a frequency of 15-22 megahertz. Essential oils have a frequency of 70-320 megahertz.

These oils oxygenate and revitalize the body. Oils also have the ability to transport nutrients and micronutrients to the body's tissues and enhance the body's energy. One example is the oil helichrysum, which when applied externally on the body improves the nervous system, stimulating the brain's synaptic firing of an electrical impulse from one nerve to another. Many of the body's functions generate and utilize electrical energy whose frequencies are measured routinely by an electrocardiogram or electroencephalogram. (These are instruments that measure the heart function and the brain waves, respectively.) The electrofrequencies can be changed by the oils. They balance and raise the energies.

Emotions Translate into the Physical

One important aspect of raising the vitality of a person is to remove negative emotional and mental patterns that they have acquired and replace them with positive, creative patterns. Until this concept is addressed fully, disease cannot be reversed completely, nor can the patient be considered completely healthy. I believe that the entire body is a totally synchronized energy machine; if there is a restriction of energy in a specific region of the body, weakness or breakdown in that area could occur.

When I began to study patterns in patients, I finally understood more about the true cause of disease and health. The negative emotions, such as fear, anger, hatred, jealousy, envy, and prejudices, suppress the spirit and, hence, the very nature of man. The person who is filled with emotions such as these is sick physically, mentally, and spiritually. For example, patients who are more "fixed" in their thought and behavior patterns often suffer from arthritis; rigidity in thoughts creates inflexibility in the body. Persons who have pent-up emotions and are under a lot of stress frequently have hypertension, which is unrelieved internal pressure. Interestingly enough, these types of patients seldom develop cancer, which instead seems to be caused by other types of behavior, such as fear of loss or loneliness. Often patients who have difficulty expressing love and other personal feelings have blocked coronary (heart) arteries. At times, these patients may feel unloved as well.

A relatively new science has emerged in which the way we think and act affects our immune system either positively or negatively. This science is called "Psychoneuroimmunology."

The whole category of immune suppression diseases has to do with a host of issues directed inwardly at the patient's life force. This creates disturbances of the immune system. We know this immune suppression is regulated by a part of the brain called the hypothalamus. It helps to modulate emotions such as joy, happiness, sadness, and anger. We understand that our environment is full of toxins and poisons. However, it is obvious that simply being exposed to these poisonous substances does not necessarily insure that disease will prevail.

Repeatedly, we physicians see several patients in the same family who are subjected to similar problems, yet may have completely different responses and outcomes. One may have a disease; the other may be totally healthy. Generally, the difference lies in their individual attitudes and behaviors. So many of our problems are the result of the inability to release old, suppressed hurts that have occurred in the past. It is these hurts that project from the subconscious as reminders of some actual or perceived injury. This injury lodges in the region of the body that most appropriately relates to the specific emotion. For instance, love has to do with the heart, breast, or bladder — the "giving" glands.

Time and time again, we are told to give up the old hurts and negative emotions. If we do not do this, these emotions clearly could manifest as disease or injury. The body literally starts taking it out on itself."

On the positive side of health, love is the purest and most important emotion that we can express. Love taken to its highest form is the most profound expression of our spiritual selves. At this elevated creation, love is called "unconditional" by some religions, while other religions refer to it as agape. Here we love fully, no matter what happens—no "ifs," "ands," or "buts." When love is openly given to others, miracles can happen.

There is a complete lack of condemnation here. We know condemnation of others, as well as self, limits health and healing and creates blocks of negative emotion. Anger, fear, and guilt are some of the most destructive emotions. These cause blocks in the natural energy flow of the body that ultimately could lead to breakdown and disease. The opposite of this is love and forgiveness, and the expression of it. Love is the most healing modality known on earth today.

What is the key for diagnosing and releasing these patterns? One effective procedure is hypnotherapy. In competent hands, this process can remove deeply established blocks. Once these blocks have been removed, healing can occur.

There are many physical reasons for a breakdown, such as hereditary weakness, nutritional deficiency, fatigue, and accidents. But they often are linked to a deeper pattern. There is a positive effect from simply recognizing the problem; that is, digging it out of the subconscious and experiencing it at a tolerable, conscious level. Releasing the problem mentally and emotionally is likely to cause the physical condition to disappear eventually. As simple as it seems, this works. Similar changes occur with homeopathic remedies, particularly if they are given at higher dilutions. If the right remedy is given, they help to remove the negative emotion.

Obviously, each person must deal with many emotions. Removing these problems one at a time is like peeling away multiple layers of an onion's skin. They unfold, one at a time, until you get down to the sweet, internal part. This healthy inner core is vibrant and complete within itself, free of illness. You have the freedom to change negative emotions any time you wish, but always do it with joy. Joy is not only a result of us achieving this balanced center, but a joyful attitude along the way helps in the process of finding that new inner peace as well.

In summary, this five step program is very comprehensive. Perhaps in some cases only a portion of the program is necessary to achieve a healthy success. With a strong immune system, we not only are able to prevent, but also to reverse disease. This applies to many diseases, such as cardiovascular diseases, allergies, multiple sclerosis, diabetes, chronic fatigue, arthritis, and cancer.

There is no need to continue to suffer from a chronic debilitating disease. This program works because it is based on firm scientific data and personal experience with these diseases in my practice. The most powerful tool we have to heal ourselves is our belief system. Either we believe in the physician and his program, or the physician must believe firmly in his ability to heal someone because of his past successes. The implication is that our degree of belief in something is a good indication as to whether or not the disease process will come to a successful and healthy conclusion.

CHAPTER 9

*Holistic Approach to
the Number One Killer
in the United States: Heart Disease*

THE BIG "H"

THE NUMBER ONE KILLER in the United States is atherosclerosis or heart disease and the resulting diseases of heart attacks and strokes. Atherosclerosis is a condition caused by hardened or calcified blood vessels. These vessels contain plaques that decrease their diameter and consequently restrict the flow of blood to cells and tissues. This results in reduced oxygen and nutrients reaching the tissues. Tissues that are undernourished are unable to function at their optimal level and, because they are malnourished, the cells become more prone to disease and even premature death.

Some warning signs of heart disease are chest pains, shortness of breath, excessive fatigue, leg pain while walking, discolored and cold feet and hands, and weakness and numbness of the arms and legs. Other signs are dizziness, light-headedness, temporary loss of vision, and impaired memory. There are many other potential symptoms not mentioned here.

🌿 What Created this Condition?

Diet

According to our past surgeon general, Dr. Julian Littmann, this condition is caused by an unhealthy life-style that includes a diet high in sugar, refined carbohydrates, and fats. Foods such as sweets, dairy products, and red meats make up the bulk of the average American diet.

Lack of exercise

Another problem is lack of exercise. Americans are notorious for riding everywhere instead of walking. They also sit for hours watching television, which offers no physical activity and encourages the increased consumption of so-called "junk foods."

Smoking and Other Pollutants

Smoking is a major risk factor for production of atherosclerosis. Many smokers complain early in life of circulatory problems in both hands and feet.

Other pollutants and toxic chemicals in our environment are very hazardous to our bodies. These include food preservatives, insecticides, and fertilizers. Also included are heavy metals such as aluminum, cadmium, and lead. Even the chlorine added to public drinking water has been linked to heart disease in some scientific studies. Keep in mind that seventy years ago in this country, heart disease was relatively unknown. This was about the period when our city water supply systems were introducing chlorine as an antibacterial agent. Bottled water is preferable for drinking.

Iron It Out!

Several years ago, a well-organized study done in Finland revealed a significant relationship between body iron and atherosclerosis. This may explain the difference in the rates of heart problems between males and females of a specific age group. Women menstruate, therefore depleting their iron stores, which could in part explain their lower rate of heart disease. Reinforcing the accuracy of this study is the fact that the frequency of heart disease in women catches up to men several years after they stop their menses.

Some sources of iron include iron water pipes, cooking in iron pots and skillets, and taking iron supplements, even when they are not needed.

Higher and Higher

Hypertension (high blood pressure) now affects up to 85 million Americans. It increases atherosclerosis by increasing the pressure and trauma to the artery wall as blood pulses through on the way to organs; micro hemorrhages are thought to occur, damaging the vessel wall.

Homocysteine

As I have said many times, the pursuit of preventive medicine is critical in obtaining good health. Therefore, I am constantly searching for new and safe modalities. The connection between a biological substance and heart disease was discovered in 1969 by Dr. Kilmer S. McCully, who was a Harvard pathologist. Dr. McCully found that a high level of the compound homocysteine in the blood stream predisposes to atherosclerosis. In his research, he evaluated an eight-year-old girl who died of heart disease due to a inherited metabolic condition that produced elevated homocysteine in her blood. The child's uncle died of a stroke, also at eight years of age. Our bodies normally make a small amount of homocysteine, but in cases where we make too much, problems can occur.

The mechanism for this pathology is as follows: Apparently, homocysteine accelerates the oxidation of cholesterol and other fats and thereby increases the rate of damage to the arteries. Antioxidants on the other hand reverse and slow this process. What accolades did Dr. McCully receive for his wisdom and innovation? None. On the contrary, his colleagues scoffed at him for his "crazy idea" and requested that he leave Harvard

Like so many medical pioneers, the "Ivy Halls Group" wear large blinders. Since the treatments for many health problems do not require a drug for which a patent can be obtained, no pharmaceutical company will invest research or grant money in a educational or investigational institute to evaluate the solution to the disease. If the "powers that be" had listened to Dr. McCully so many years ago and adapted his simple program, perhaps thousands of lives could have been saved. This points out the medical profession's bias against any pioneering physicians who do independent research and claim success with their patients.

The nutrients that reverse elevated homocysteine levels, through the interference of its increased production by abnormal body metabolism, are antioxidants and vitamins. The nutrients successfully used are vitamins B_{12} (cyanocobalmin), B6 (pyridoxine) and folic acid.

The doses for vitamin B_{12} are, 100-1000 mcg daily; vitamin B6, 50 -100 mg daily, best taken at night; and folic acid, approximately 400 mcg daily, depending on the severity of the condition. These products are water soluble and are considered very safe as they are not easily stored in excessive amounts. They are recommended for everyone but particularly if you have elevated homocysteine blood levels. Since homocysteine is accepted as a risk factor in the cause of atherosclerosis today, one should have a blood test measuring the levels of homocysteine. This is especially true if you have a high family incidence of heart disease or if you are over 40 years of age. Simple precaution may save your life.

All Stressed Out
Stress is another precursor to atherosclerosis. Certain biochemical and hormonal reactions occur during an unpleasant encounter. The mechanism of plaque formation is accelerated unless steps are taken to reduce this. We are all aware that in this busy society the degree of stress has been increasing during the last half of this century.

❦ DIAGNOSIS

The following tests may be performed to diagnose and measure circulatory problems: Doppler studies of the neck and extremities using sound waves; angiography, a method in which dye is injected in the arteries while x-rays are being taken; blood tests; cardiac stress tests; and the new ultra-fast CAT scan of the arteries. Some of these tests, such as angiography, are very expensive and carry health risks.

Current Procedures and Fixes

Once the diagnosis of atherosclerosis has been made, what do we do to correct the situation?

Billions of dollars are spent annually on health care in this country, much of it on problems of atherosclerosis. With heart and coronary disease, a procedure called bypass surgery is quite often recommended. This is a very expensive procedure that has a high risk of complications—from 0.5 to 10 percent depending upon where the surgery is performed. The morbidity rate is much higher.

During the last several years a procedure called angioplasty has been developed. In this procedure, the doctor opens the arteries by inserting a catheter and inflating a balloon while inside the artery. This exerts pressure on the plaque, actually crushing it into the wall of the artery, thereby opening the passage. This too has risk of causing injury or death, but not nearly as much as bypass surgery.

Another technique is a reaming procedure in which the inside of the artery is cored out like an apple. Again, this procedure has considerable associated risk.

One of the latest procedures is the use of a cold laser to vaporize the plaque within the vessel. Also called cold laser, it is used to burn channels into the heart, which eventually opens up new circulation. This procedure appears to have great promise. However, there are very few physicians in the country who are trained in coronary laser therapy.

In the case of strokes, one cause is the blockage of the carotid arteries in the neck by atherosclerotic plaque. Surgically, these may be opened and the plaque stripped out. There is a risk in this procedure. The other problem is that other cerebral vessels that nourish the brain also become blocked and could produce strokes. Unfortunately, they are much more difficult to reach than the carotid artery. In fact, it is virtually impossible to surgically remove plaque from most of these arteries.

Problems with Surgical Procedures

The problem with all of these surgical procedures is that the artery tends to reblock in approximately 50 percent of the cases. Unfortunately, the block may reoccur in as little six weeks. Another problem with these procedures is that they are very expensive, costing from $10,000 to $75,000 per procedure on average. It can even run much more if complications develop and the hospital stay is extended.

In addition the atherosclerosis is present throughout the circulatory system, while the treatment is obviously localized and limited to the small region, an inch or so in length, that is addressed with these procedures. That leaves the rest of the body, literally many miles of arteries, untreated and ignored by most physicians. In fact it is possible for a patient to have a stroke while on the operating table having bypass surgery.

THE HOLISTIC ANSWER

The holistic physician has another answer; it is called chelation (pronounced key-lay-shun). Chelation is safe, effective, and compared to other procedures, a relatively inexpensive treatment. It restores, without surgery, the blood flow in victims of atherosclerosis.

Chelation therapy involves the intravenous infusion (injected directly into a blood vessel) of a compound called ethylene diamine tetra-acetic acid (EDTA). This substance removes undesirable metals and minerals from the body. Many of these metals—lead, mercury, cadmium, and aluminum—are poisons. Aluminum is currently believed to be a major contributor to Alzheimer's disease. You can accumulate aluminum from antacids, under arm deodorants, canned drinks, and aluminum cookware. Other metals and minerals, such as iron, mercury, and calcium, may be destructive as well. Some are harmless in small amounts, but in excess may be deposited in the organs of the body and around the joints as well as within the blood vessels.

Many heavy metals, ultraviolet radiation, fats, and pollution in general cause damage to cell membranes by producing "oxygen free radicals." All tissues contain building blocks called atoms, which are orbited by electrons. These atoms normally combine to form molecules, which in turn make up tissues. Under normal circumstances these elements are stable. But when they are exposed to these damaging elements they may lose one of their electrons and become unstable. They will then steal electrons from surrounding tissue, and a chain reactions of electron swapping may occur. This reaction is a form of oxidation (gone wild) and causes serious cellular damage. This process plays a central role in the aging process as well as in the progression of disease and, ultimately, cellular death.

Free radical pathology is now believed by many scientists to be an important contributory cause of atherosclerosis, cancer, diabetes, and other diseases of aging. EDTA helps to prevent the production of free radicals. It also removes them once they are established. Usually a minimum of thirty chelation treatments is recommended.

As evidence that chelation therapy is among the safest of medical procedures, more than 500,000 patients have received over five million treatments during the last thirty years. To my knowledge, not one death has been directly caused by chelation therapy when properly administered. Of course, it must be administered by a physician who is fully trained and competent in the use of this therapy.

A meta-analysis (a study of studies) has been published. It shows a highly statistical probability that chelation leads to improvement as demonstrated by objective testing. In this study of 22,765 patients, 87 percent demonstrated measurable improvement in their circulation between pre- and post-treatment testing.

In the country of New Zealand, the government passed a law making it illegal to be subjected to bypass surgery until chelation therapy has been tried. Undoubtedly, this is because chelation is much less expensive, is certainly a safer procedure, and has a higher "lasting" success rate.

One of the most important aspects of chelation is the use of this modality for prevention. Since it has been shown that the process of atherosclerosis begins as early as the teenage years, then a program to reverse this at the early stages must be considered.

In cases in which there has been damage to the heart muscle itself, chelation offers a possible solution. There are frequently muscle cells of the heart that are not dead but are dormant or otherwise operating in a reduced manner due to poor capillary or other circulation problems. Chelation can often clear this problem, offering a renewal of the tissues as well as renewal of life for the patient.

Cross Section of a Blood Vessel

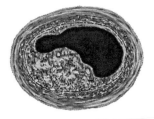 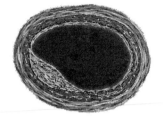

Before Chelation Therapy   *After Chelation Therapy*

In the case of stroke, chelation has much to offer. As an example, in the early stages chelation may reverse damage to the brain. By rapidly removing free radicals that form during a stroke and improving the circulation, damage may be reduced and recovery time accelerated. I have seen some strokes actually stopped in process by utilizing chelation very early on in the process.

Diet and Exercise

Along with chelation, one must make other life-style changes. Not only should one avoid habits such as smoking, but one must follow a low-fat, salt, and sugar diet, and exercise regularly, thereby keeping weight in the normal range.

Keep in mind that dairy products are high in fat and should be excluded as much as possible. Also dairy products have a mucus substance in their makeup. This has a serious deleterious effect in that it causes a stickiness in the blood, interfering with the normal flow. So although a patient may choose low-fat products, if they are sticky they may be dangerous over time. It appears that the detrimental affects are noted on adults and not children. Look to nature for examples. You never see adult cows (or any other animals) drinking milk after they have been weaned.

I specifically stress a diet that includes fish, particularly salmon, because it is rich in highly unsaturated fatty acids of the omega-3 family. These assist in reducing blood cholesterol. I also tell my patients to reduce or, better yet, eliminate red meats and pork, and to eat chicken only occasionally. I encourage eating lots of fresh vegetables, preferably organically grown. I add some, but not large amounts, of fresh fruits to the diet. (Too much fruit is not good, in my opinion, because it contains a large amount of sugar, even though it is fruit sugar.) Next I include whole grains, namely oats, millet, barley, amaranth, and rice. Wheat is to be eaten only if the patient has no history of allergies, and then must be limited to whole grain. For pasta, I emphasize Jerusalem artichoke pasta, found in most health food stores. All cooked foods should be prepared by boiling, broiling, baking, or stir frying, using little fat and then only olive, safflower, canola, or a similar polyunsaturated oil.

Next, I tell my patients that it is essential that they take supplements. First I include a multivitamin and mineral, extra Vitamin C, E, and B6. Then I add Ginkgo Biloba to improve alertness and circulation, coenzyme Q-10 for extra energy and oxygen, and flax seed oil with omega-3, 6's, and 9's or fish oils. These oils are high in the polyunsaturated fat (the good kind), which is made up of three helpful oils called omega-3, linoleic acid, made up of alpha linolenic, oleic, eiocosapentaenoic acid, and docosahexaenoic acid. While these are the basic supplements, there are other helpful ones, but they are added because of specific problems. I design a supplement plan for each patient.

I encourage my patients to add to this a healthier life-style and a reduction in stress. If these guidelines are followed, a chelation therapy program designed for persons of adult age could prolong the length and improve the quality of life.

❧ Beneficial Side Effects

With chelation, the toxic heavy metals—lead, mercury, cadmium, and aluminum, as well as excess iron and calcium—are removed from the tissues. I have observed the improved function of many organs, including the kidneys (even in cases of mild kidney failure), after chelation. I have also noted leg pain with exercise disappearing and cardiac angina being alleviated. A number of patients have declared that their eyesight as well as memory and general energy level have improved. Many patients have also reported that their fingernails have gotten stronger and grown faster, and that normal color has returned to their gray hair. They are more youthful in both action and appearance.

❧ A Case of Sensitivity

There are other chelating agents. A couple of years ago, my patient, Steve, was a successful practicing dentist. He was middle-aged and had everything that middle-class Americans strive for: a wonderful wife and two children, a station wagon, and a beautiful house on the lake. He belonged to the country club and enjoyed playing golf every week. Steve was seemingly healthy and did not lack for much.

Then one day Steve's life began to change. He started to experience headaches, light-headedness, and uneasiness in his chest. Initially these symptoms occurred occasionally and did not last long. Then they became more frequent, occurring daily and then several times a day, lasting for hours. He became concerned and sought professional help. Because he was a professional himself, he got plenty of advice from his colleagues.

However, in spite of their good intentions, Steve rapidly became worse, experiencing a pounding and racing heart, chest pain, diarrhea, insomnia, sweats, aching joints, and, worst of all, anxiety and panic attacks. He began missing work and his patients complained that he didn't look well and seemed inattentive, irritable, and indifferent. They were concerned and frequently mentioned it to his nurse.

By this time, his family was alarmed about his personality changes and his wife suggested he seek psychiatric counseling because he was beginning to experience an inability to concentrate, along with confusion and persistent depression. Steve took her advice and went to a psychiatrist, who prescribed a strong antidepressant. Within one week, not only were his symptoms worse but he had some new ones. He complained of skin rashes and itching, excessive drowsiness, nausea, vomiting, and extreme weakness and fatigue. He was then referred to other specialists including a cardiologist, a dermatologist, and an endocrinologist, with each recommending his own brand of drugs and/or therapy. All this occurred within a couple of months from the onset of the original symptoms. He was missing a great deal of work, finding it hard to get up and started each morning. Then, at the advice of his psychiatrist, Steve entered the hospital for a thorough checkup that included a digestive exam, a complete heart evaluation, and an endocrine study.

The results of the exam did not reveal anything unusual. All during this time, not suspecting a common denominator, his respective specialists gave him more medications. One drug was for depression, another for anxiety, and others for heart, stomach, and so forth. He felt much worse in general, even after getting out of the hospital. Steve was barely functioning by now and spent most of his time lying around the house, and he still didn't have an idea as to the diagnosis. He did observe one thing about himself, however; he seemed to feel worse at his dental office.

One day, after discussing the situation with his wife, he decided to close down his dental practice and attempt to live temporarily on the little savings he had until he felt good enough to go back to work. One thing kept reoccurring in his mind, however. He had read an article in some dental magazine regarding the existence of a rare occurrence of a sensitivity to mercury. Mercury is used by dentists in preparation of silver amalgam fillings, the most common type of filling used in the United States today. Some of the symptoms mentioned in the article were similar to the ones he exhibited.

About this time, Steve heard about my work with patients suffering from severe allergic problems, including sensitivity to heavy metals and chemicals. After a complete evaluation, it was determined that he indeed had multiple sensitivities to his environment that were triggered by three significant events occurring approximately one month before Steve had his first symptom. First, he had experienced a very frustrating and traumatic family situation that caused him both anxiety and anger. He was unable to resolve this situation or to deal with his emotional feelings. Second, his dental technician became ill and he had to do his own amalgam preparation. Third, that week, his air conditioner broke down and he became faint while mixing the amalgam in a small, stuffy laboratory room with no ventilation.

It is now known that minute amounts of mercury vapor are given off from these amalgam fillings, whether being mixed by a technician or after they have been in the mouth for some time. This mercury ultimately finds its way into the blood stream where it is carried to the nervous system. Mercury has an affinity for the nerves, and the term "mad as a hatter," which was coined a century ago, comes from the fact that hat makers then used a substance called "quick silver," or mercury, to block top hats. These people often became psychotic after years of working with mercury that eventually accumulated in their brains. Mercury is also found in the liver, kidneys, and the lining of the intestinal tract.

However, the mercury also stressed the immune systems of people who were sensitive to its effects. According to some data, as many as 1 percent of the population is in this category today. That represents over 2½ million people. However, I feel that the actual percentage is much higher. The American Dental Association has taken the stand that mercury sensitivity is rare and does not constitute a serious problem. Nevertheless, numerous people seem to improve in health and vitality once these amalgams are removed.

The tests done on Steve revealed that he had a leakage of mercury from some of his amalgam fillings; after their removal he felt somewhat better. He was then placed on a complete detoxification and regeneration program. He was administered a mercury chelating agent called DMPS. This removes the mercury from the tissues and eliminates it by way of the kidneys. In other words, you urinate the metal out.

Steve slowly began to regain his health, energy, and normal functioning. It was a long process for him, however. But, eventually he was able to return to his practice.

✂ SYNDROME "X"

Many people that suffer from a cardiovascular disease have a condition that promotes it called Syndrome "X." It is estimated that 10 to 15 percent of the population has this genetic tendency. Sufferers have a high LDL fat, which is damaging to the blood vessels. Their total cholesterol is also elevated significantly above 200. They have high triglycerides, which is the milky white fat carried by the blood.

Another problem that accompanies this condition is insulin resistance. This means that if the patient consumes simple carbohydrates or sugars, instead of making them into insulin to lower the blood sugar, the body does not respond to insulin. This causes the body to make more and more insulin in an internal attempt to control the sugar. It will finally perform its action, but not until a high level of insulin is found in the body. This high level of insulin does further damage to the blood vessels.

Some of the symptoms of Syndrome "X" are elevated blood sugar and high blood pressure. This condition may lead to premature stroke and heart attack. Treatment includes maintaining a normal weight, getting regular exercise, and eating a proper diet, along with chelation therapy. The correct diet would be to reduce saturated fats and simple sugars.

☙ SUMMARY

In summary, chelation is a safe effective method of removing excess calcium, lead, and other unwanted deleterious products from the body. It should be tried in all suspected cases of atherosclerosis.

Unfortunately, chelation is not generally known about or understood by the mainstream medical community today. One often hears from other physicians that there is no published evidence confirming the efficacy of chelation therapy. This is surprising considering that there is much published data confirming these facts. Consequently, I have included over thirty references involving cases of persons, most of whom have benefited from chelation therapy. This list, appearing at the end of this chapter, is just a small sampling of the documentation dealing with chelation therapy.

☙ SUGGESTED READING

The following are books on chelation therapy that I strongly recommend to anyone that has atherosclerosis, heart disease, or *angina pectoris*, or to anyone contemplating any type of invasive cardiovascular or vascular procedure:

Brecher, Harold, and Arline Brecher. *Forty Something Forever: A Consumer's Guide to Chelation Therapy and Other Heart-Savers.* Herndon, VA: Healthsavers Press, 1992.

Cranton, Elmer, M.D., and Arline Brecher. *Bypassing Bypass.* Herndon, VA: Medex Press, 1984. (Contains 233 additional references.)

Julian, James J., M.D. *Chelation Extends Life.* Hollywood, CA: Wellness Press, 1982. (Contains 25 additional references.)

McDonagh, E.W., D.O. *Chelation Can Cure.* Kansas City, MO: Platinum Pen Publishers, 1983. (Contains 78 additional references.)

Quinn, Dick. *Left for Dead.* Minneapolis, MN: R.F. Quinn Publishing Co., 1992. (Contains 49 additional references.)

REFERENCES

Bjorksten, Johan, PhD. "The Crosslinkage Theory of Aging as a Predictive Indicator," from *Rejuvenation, The Official Journal of the International Association on the Artifficial Prolongation of the Human Specific Lifespan.* Belgium, 1979. (Contains 169 additional references.)

_____. "Possibilities and Limitations of Chelation as a Means for Life Extension," from *Rejuvenation, The Official Journal of the International Association on the Artifficial Prolongation of the Human Specific Lifespan.* Belgium, 1979. (Contains 43 additional references).

Blumer, Walter, MD, and Elmer M. Cranton, MD. "Ninety Percent Reduction in Cancer Mortality after Chelation Therapy with EDTA," from *Journal of Advancement in Medicine,* Spring/Summer 1989, Vol. 2, Nos. 1/2. New York: Human Sciences Press, Inc. (Contains 26 additional references.)

Carter, James P., MD, DrPH. "If EDTA Chelation Therapy Is So Good, Why Is It Not More Widely Accepted?," from *Journal of Advancement in Medicine,* Spring/Summer 1989, Vol. 2, Nos. 1/2. New York: Human Sciences Press, Inc. (Contains 11 additional references.)

Casdorph, H. Richard, MD. "EDTA Chelation Therapy: Efficacy in Arteriosclerotic Heart Disease," from *Journal of Advancement in Medicine,* Spring/Summer 1989, Vol. 2, Nos. 1/2. New York: Human Sciences Press, Inc. (Contains 16 additional references.)

_____. "EDTA Chelation Therapy: Efficacy in Brain Disorders," from *Journal of Advancement in Medicine,* Spring/Summer 1989, Vol. 2, Nos. 1/2. New York: Human Sciences Press, Inc. (Contains 18 additional references.)

Cheraskin, Emanuel, MD, DMD, Doug G. Wussow, Edward W. McDonagh, DO, FACGP, and Charles J. Rudolph, DO, PhD. "Effect of EDTA Chelation and Supportive Multivitamin/Trace Mineral Supplementation with and without Physical Activity on the Heart Rate," from *The Journal of the Inter-*

national Academy of Preventive Medicine, November, 1984. (Contains 18 additional references.)

Cranton, Elmer M., MD. "A Textbook on EDTA Chelation Therapy," from *Journal of Advancement in Medicine,* Spring/Summer 1989, Vol. 2, Nos. 1/2. New York: Human Sciences Press, Inc. (Contains 11 additional references.)

_____. "Protocol of the American College of Advancement in Medicine for the Safe and Effective Administration of EDTA Chelation Therapy," from *Journal of Advancement in Medicine,* Spring/Summer 1989, Vol. 2, Nos. 1/2. New York: Human Sciences Press, Inc. (Contains 119 additional references.)

_____. "Kidney Effects of Ethylene Diamine Tetraacetic Acid (EDTA): A Literature Review," from *Journal of Advancement in Medicine,* Spring/Summer 1989, Vol. 2, Nos. 1/2. New York: Human Sciences Press, Inc. (Contains 31 additional references.)

_____. "Interpretation of Trace and Toxic Element Levels in Human Hair," from *Journal of Advancement in Medicine,* Spring/Summer 1989, Vol. 2, Nos. 1/2. New York: Human Sciences Press, Inc. (Contains 169 additional references.)

Cranton, Elmer M., MD, and James P. Frackelton, MD. "Free Radical Pathology in Age-Associated Diseases: Treatment with EDTA Chelation, Nutrition, and Antioxidants," from *Journal of Advancement in Medicine,* Spring/Summer 1989, Vol. 2, Nos. 1/2. New York: Human Sciences Press, Inc. (Contains 232 additional references.)

_____. "Current Status of EDTA Chelation Therapy in Occlusive Arterial Disease," from *Journal of Advancement in Medicine,* Spring/Summer 1989, Vol. 2, Nos. 1/2. New York: Human Sciences Press, Inc. (Contains 37 additional references.)

Cranton, Elmer M., MD, Zheng Xian Liu, MS, and Ivy M. Smith, MT. "Urinary Trace and Toxic Elements and Minerals in Untimed Urine Specimens Relative to Urine Creatinine, Part I: Concentrations of Elements in Fasting Urine," from *Journal of Advancement in Medicine,* Spring/Summer 1989, Vol. 2, Nos. 1/2. New York: Human Sciences Press, Inc. (Contains 11 additional references.)

_____. "Urinary Trace and Toxic Elements and Minerals in Untimed Urine Specimens Relative to Urine Creatinine, Part II: Provoked Increase in Excretion Following Intravenous EDTA," from *Journal of Advancement in Medicine,* Spring/Summer 1989, Vol. 2, Nos. 1/2. New York: Human Sciences Press, Inc. (Contains 9 additional references.)

Frackelton, James P. MD. "Monitoring Renal Function During EDTA Chelation Therapy," from *Journal of Advancement in Medicine*, Spring/Summer 1989, Vol. 2, Nos. 1/2. New York: Human Sciences Press, Inc. (Contains 6 additional references.)

Frackelton, James P. MD, and Elmer M. Cranton, MD. "Iron and Copper Supplementation with EDTA Chelation Therapy," presented at the Third Annual German Congress on Chelation Therapy, Munich, March 1, 1986. (Contains 12 additional references.)

Gaby, Alan R., MD. "Nutritional Factors in Cardiovascular Disease," from *Journal of Advancement in Medicine*, Spring/Summer 1989, Vol. 2, Nos. 1/2. New York: Human Sciences Press, Inc. (Contains 99 additional references.)

McDonagh, E.W., DO, FACGP, Charles J. Rudolph, DO, PhD, and Emanuel Cheraskin, MD, DMD. "An Oculocerebrovasculometric Analysis of the Improvement in Arterial Stenosis Following EDTA Chelation Therapy," from *Journal of Advancement in Medicine*, Spring/Summer 1989, Vol. 2, Nos. 1/2. New York: Human Sciences Press, Inc. (Contains 6 additional references.)

_____. "The Effect of EDTA Chelation Therapy Plus Supportive Multivitamin-Trace Mineral Supplementation Upon Renal Function: A Study in Serum Creatinine," from *Journal of Advancement in Medicine*, Spring/Summer 1989, Vol. 2, Nos. 1/2. New York: Human Sciences Press, Inc. (Contains 3 additional references.)

_____. "The 'Clinical Change' in Patients Treated with EDTA Chelation Plus Multivitamin/Trace Mineral Supplementation," from *Journal of Orthomolecular Psychiatry*, Vol. 14, 1985. (Contains 22 additional references.)

_____. "The Effect of EDTA Chelation Therapy Plus Supportive Multivitamin-Trace Mineral Supplementation UponRenal Function: A Study in Blood Urea Nitrogen (BUN)," from *Journal of Advancement in Medicine*, Spring/Summer 1989, Vol. 2, Nos. 1/2. New York: Human Sciences Press, Inc. (Contains 3 additional references.)

_____. "Serum Cholesterol and the Aging Process," from *Medical Hypotheses*, 7: 685-694, 1981. (Contains 15 additional references.)

_____. "The Homeostatic Effect of EDTA with Supportive Multivitamin Trace Mineral Supplementation Upon High-Density Lipoproteins (HDL)," from *The Journal of the Osteopathic Physicians and Surgeons of California*, 8:2, Spring Issue 1982. (Contains 3 additional references.)

_____. "The Effect of Intravenous Disodium Ethylene Diamine Tetraacetic Acid (EDTA) upon Blood Cholesterol in a Private Practice Environment," from *The Journal of the International Academy of Preventive Medicine*, Vol. VII:1, April, 1982. (Contains 10 additional references.)

_____. "The Glycohemoglobin (HbAlc) Distribution in EDTA-Chelation-Eligible Patients," from *The Journal of Orthomolecular Psychiatry*, Vol. 12:1. (Contains 7 additional references.)

_____. "The Influence of EDTA Salts Plus Multivitamin-Trace Mineral Therapy Upon Total Serum Cholesterol/High-Density Lipoprotein Cholesterol," from *Medical Hypotheses*, 9: 643-646, 1982. (Contains 7 additional references.)

_____. "The Nutrition-Prevention Connection," from *Osteopathic Annals*, p. 109-115, 1983. (Contains 6 additional references.)

_____. "The Effect of EDTA Chelation Therapy with Multivitamin/Trace Mineral Supplementation Upon Reported Fatigue," from *The Journal of Orthomolecular Psychiatry*, Vol. 13, No. 4. (Contains 3 additional references.)

_____. "The Psychotherapeutic Potential of EDTA Chelation," from *The Journal of Orthomolecular Psychiatry*, Vol. 14, No. 3. (Contains 11 additional references.)

_____. "The Effect of Intravenous Disodium Ethylene Diamine Tetraacetic Acid (EDTA) Plus Supportive Multivitamin/Trace Mineral Supplementation Upon Fasting Serum Calcium," from *Medical Hypotheses*, 11: 431-438. (Contains 13 additional references.)

Olszewer, Efrain, MD, and James P. Carter, MD, DrPH. "EDTA Chelation Therapy: A Retrospective Study of 2,870 Patients," from *Medical Hypotheses*, 1988, Vol. 27, pages 41-49. New Orleans: Churchill Livingstone Publishers. (Contains 27 additional references.)

Passwater, Richard, MD, and Elmer M. Cranton, MD. *Trace Elements, Hair Analysis and Nutrition.* New Canaan, CT: Keats Publishing Co., 1983.

Riordan, Hugh D., MD, Emanuel Cheraskin, MD, DMD, Marvin Dirks, BD, MA, Mavis Schultz, ARNP, and Penny Brizendine, ARNP. "Another Look at Renal Function and the EDTA Chelation Treatment Process," from *Journal of Orthomolecular Medicine*, Vol 2, 1987. (Contains 6 additional references.)

Rudolph, Charles J., Jr., DO, PhD. "Trace Element Patterning in Degenerative Diseases," from *The Journal of the International Academy of Preventive Medicine*, July, 1977. (Contains 33 additional references.)

Rudolph, Charles J. Jr., DO, PhD, Edward W. McDonagh, DO, FACGP, FAPM. "The Chelation Carrier Solution: An Analysis of Osmolarity and Sodium Content," from *Journal of the International Academy of Preventive Medicine*, Vol. VIII, No. 1, Winter, 1983. (Contains 14 additional references.)

Sehnert, Keith W., MD, A.F. Clague, and Emanuel Cheraskin, MD, DMD. "The Improvement in Renal Function Following EDTA Chelation and

Multivitamin-Trace Mineral Therapy: A Study in Creatinine Clearance,"
from *Medical Hypotheses*, Vol. 15, 1984. Minneapolis: Churchill Livingstone
Publishers. (Contains 11 additional references.)

Sullivan, Jerome L., MD, PhD. "Iron and Ischemic Heart Disease,"
from *Journal of Advancement in Medicine*, Spring/Summer 1989, Vol. 2, Nos.
1/2. New York: Human Sciences Press, Inc. (Contains 27 additional references.)

CHAPTER 10

Allergies and the Immune System

TIP OF THE ICEBERG

ALLERGIES AND DISEASES of the immune system should be considered the diseases of the 21st century. Scientists estimate that approximately 25 percent of the U.S. population suffers to some degree from allergies alone; however, other clinicians feel the actual number is much higher. However, even this figure represents 58 million people.

Today we are just seeing the tip of the iceberg as it relates to these diseases that, unfortunately, are being experienced by more and more people. The problems of allergies and low immunity cause much suffering for those who are either not receiving proper diagnoses or not even seeking help from a physician. These diseases are more prevalent today than they were just a few years ago because we are being subjected to increasingly large numbers of chemicals and exotic foods with preservatives. Subsequently we are also accumulating these substances in our bodies.

The definition of allergies was given by Clemon Von Pinquet in 1906. He combined two Greek words, allos, meaning "other," and ergon, meaning "action." Therefore, an allergic person reacts to substances that do not affect other people.

More recently, other terms such as "sensitivity," "hypersensitive," and "maladaptive reaction," have been used in place of the word "allergy." This is because certain foods and other allergens do not evoke the typical antigen-antibody response that is commonly seen in allergies in which the body defends itself against foreign substances. This is not to be confused with food intolerance, which means that our body systems are unable to digest, absorb, or utilize certain foods.

There are four basic ways in which we may experience allergic reactions: through substances that we breathe, through substances that we eat and drink, through substances that are in direct contact with our skin, and through substances such as drugs and toxins that are injected into the body. We may be allergic or sensitive in one or more of these ways.

Some people have multiple sensitivities to substances from the external environment and manifest a syndrome called "ecological illness." This field is called "clinical ecology" and deals with the individual's relationship to his or her environment.

The term "immune" comes from the Latin word immunist, which means "exempt from, resistant to, or protected from disease or infectious organisms, poisons, allergens and other agents." Our bodies tend to defend themselves against an outside substance or particle that is foreign to it.

A true allergic reaction is one that is immunologically mediated, meaning that the person has been exposed to a foreign substance, or antigen. In response to an antigen, the body sends out an antibody that attacks the foreign substance, defending the body and therefore counteracting the effect of that foreign substance.

The byproduct of the body's chemical defense reaction is called histamine. Unfortunately, an excess of histamine in the body causes tissue damage that may include swelling of the mucosal lining of the nose and throat with accompanying edema (a swelling or accumulation of fluid) and congestion of these tissues. Other possible tissue damage includes swelling and edema of intestinal mucosal that interferes with the proper absorption of food and may also produce abdominal cramping, pain, and diarrhea.

In response to stressors (anything causing stress), both physical—

chemicals, bacteria, viruses, foods, pollens, or molds — and psychological, the brain releases various substances that assist in the protection of the body.

We have two types of cells that generally react with allergens. These are T cells and B cells, both a type of antibody. In regards to allergies, we are involved with three classes of antibodies: IgG, IgM, IgE. These are just technical terms used to define different types of allergic reactions, and I will describe them as we continue.

When the T cell is the mediator (arbitrator or go-between), then we experience a dermal or skin reaction, an inflammation caused by direct contact. We can also find this type of reaction with an inflammation of the lungs leading to pneumonitis secondary to hypersensitivity to an allergen.

Regarding the IgE mediated allergic reaction, the mast cell releases histamine. The consequence of this is to produce dilation of blood vessels along with mucus secretion. These mast cells are the cause of much of the discomfort during these allergic episodes.

The immune system is stimulated by way of the thymus gland and the bursal equivalent. Products are formed whose function is to counteract the effects of the stressors.

The foreign substances, or antigens, may be plant pollens, fungal spores, insects, feathers, airborne gases and chemicals, foods, food additives, preservatives, and drugs. Others of importance are gasoline fumes, cosmetics, detergents, nylons, paints, insecticides, fertilizers, air smog or pollution, heavy metals, newspaper ink, common ink, felt-tip pens, and plastics.

✺ AIRBORNE AGENTS

Airborne agents that produce respiratory-type allergies exist worldwide. However, some areas have more while others have fewer allergy-producing substances. For example, in some large cities, such as Los Angeles, heavy amounts of certain gases and chemicals are found in the atmosphere that are mainly the result of the combustion of petroleum in the automobile. One may experience asthma, wheezing, and shortness of breath, as well as bronchitis or even emphysema, all of which are the result of long-term exposure to pollutants.

Because of the need to be economical in response to the control of our energy fuel, many newer buildings are designed to be air-tight. Consequently, because of the mechanics of this closed system, many pollutants are trapped inside. The air-conditioning ducts contain mold spores that are blown into the air. Additionally, if the environment becomes warm and moist, many other organisms have an affinity for this and generally multiply. An example is bacteria that may not only cause a respiratory infection but may also provoke an allergic reaction in many people. Therefore, the inhabitants in the entire building may be affected, one way or another, by these organisms.

House dust and animal dander, along with plant pollen and spores found floating in the air, are a source of trouble to the respiratory tract of some individuals. Others are sensitive to insects, or even insect parts that may be carried airborne by indoor dust particles and affect the respiratory system. This scenario certainly reinforces the value of fresh air and sunshine in promoting good health.

Respiratory reactions may be serious. A person may have a severe allergic reaction to airborne substances that cause difficulty in breathing and swelling around the vocal cords. This may lead to respiratory distress and heart stoppage that, if prolonged, could result in death.

Other more minor but very annoying allergic reactions are: watery nasal discharge; itching of the eyes, ears, nose, and throat; sneezing; and nasal congestion. These reactions are generally found in the condition called "hay fever." Prolonged suffering may lead to post-nasal drip, sore throat, watery eyes, bloody nose, nasal twang, snoring, and chronic mouth breathing. The symptoms often make the individual miserable and interfere with his or her normal life pattern. Blockage of the ear canals could result in chronic infection, possibly leading to deafness. Chronic blockage of the sinuses could lead to head and facial pain and sinusitis. Hay fever may be largely seasonal, but in some instances, it is experienced year 'round.

🌸 ANTIGENS INTRODUCED INTO THE BODY

Another source of antigens is drugs and other substances that are injected through the skin, including insect secretions from a sting or a bite. Sometimes the result is minor. Sometimes the substance is carried to distant parts of the body where it may create numerous problems, including respiratory compromise or serious breathing problems, and may even end in death.

🌸 FOOD ALLERGIES

Food allergy is a fascinating topic and yet is a condition that is difficult to diagnose, as shown by the following case history.

Jennie was a 32-year-old housewife with one child. She was active in the P.T.A. and a tennis club. Her hobby was painting. She led what would be considered a normal life until one day her husband came home and told her he had been transferred to Florida. Within the month, they moved. This was very emotionally traumatic for Jennie as this necessitated her leaving her friends and relatives in the Midwest.

At first she did not like Florida because of the loneliness she experienced from missing her friends and relatives. In addition, she had an aversion to insects and she was confronted immediately with large palmetto bugs in the old house they bought. It was located near the water and had been closed up for nearly a year before she and her family moved into it. She had frequently ordered the pest control people over to spray chemicals inside the house.

After living in Florida for about a month, Jennie began to complain of fatigue. This was followed by frequent periods of feeling blue and being deeply depressed. Then came frequent "crying jags." Next, her husband observed that she was much more argumentative. They had numerous arguments, some of which ended with her screaming. She gained weight rapidly and also complained of sleepiness. Her husband also noticed her lethargy and noted that after eating, she became very sleepy and often took a nap. Every time they went to a restaurant, she wanted to return home immediately after eating to sleep. She also complained that many foods distressed her. Many times, shortly after eating, she experienced nausea, bloating, belching, flatulence (passing gas), and diarrhea.

She came to my office at the insistence of her husband who was certain she had a stomach ulcer. The first thing I noticed were dark circles under Jennie's eyes. These are called "shiners" by allergists and are found in persons who have significant allergies.

After taking a comprehensive history, I found some other interesting facts about Jennie. First, as a child, she had had eczema, a skin rash, and many food allergies. She also had recurrent ear infections and tonsillitis and was prescribed antibiotics repeatedly. She eventually had her tonsils removed. She was also very allergic to insect stings and often received cortisone because the bites caused her to swell up and become short of breath. She had recurrent episodes of poison ivy that required even more cortisone injections. In her twenties, she began to have recurrent vaginitis and her gynecologist told her that this was due to candida, a yeast infection. (See Chapter 14.)

At the time of her consultation with me, she claimed that she barely finished a meal before she experienced fatigue and sleepiness. I immediately started her work-up and she was tested for food allergies and, out of more than 200 foods tested, she was allergic to sixty-eight, a very high number. It was obvious that she had developed extensive food sensitivities that, in turn, caused the sleepiness and other symptoms such as her aggressive behavior and digestive complaints. The difference between fatigue and sleepiness caused by food allergies and those caused by a low blood sugar reaction is that allergies can cause an immediate reaction while a low blood sugar reaction occurs from 1 to 3 hours after eating.

Although Jennie had a previous history of food allergies, her immune system was impaired further, until she was now unable to cope with many foods that she could consume before. For example, as a child she was allergic to many things. Since many foods were not identified and eliminated from her diet at that time, she initially developed what is known as "masked sensitivities." That means she daily ate foods to which she was allergic. In fact, she craved those foods that represented a food addiction. As long as she was subjected to small amounts of these addictive foods, there was very little overt reaction. Of course, Jennie always complained of excessive fatigue. Frequently she also experienced a mild charge of nervous energy after she ate certain foods. Unfortunately, this reaction was followed by a period of fatigue and depression.

Other events that challenged her immune system were the stress of leaving her friends and moving to Florida and the bug extermination chemicals that remained in the house and her environment for along period of time. Some of these chemicals are thought to deactivate the process of the detoxifying reaction of the liver, needed to protect us. In her youth she had often taken antibiotics and cortisone, which many experts believe depress the immune system, especially if given repeatedly, year after year.

The old house that Jennie moved into quite likely contained mold as it had been closed up for a long period of time and Florida tends to be humid. All of these factors challenged and weakened Jennie's immune system, leading to her inability to cope with food allergies.

My therapy for Jennie was a complete, comprehensive allergic treatment program that I will discuss under treatment of allergies, later in this chapter. Fortunately, Jennie responded very well to this therapy.

❦ How Allergies Develop

A rather complex mechanism is involved with the development of food allergies. The most appropriate theory is quite interesting.

The gastrointestinal (G.I.) tract may be overgrown with pathological organisms such as the bacteria Klebsiella, coxsackie enteroviruses, or fungus or protozoal microbes such as Cryptosporidium parvum or Entamoeba histolytica. These organisms may damage the inner lining of the G.I. tract or mucosa.

Certain foods can do similar damage. For example, cow's milk protein or wheat can stimulate enteropathy or damage to the G.I. tract through an activation of associated immunity reactions in cells of mucosa. As a result of these foods and those organisms described above as well as many more, the G.I. mucosa lining may be so badly damaged that one may have an altered G.I. mucosal permeability, or "Leaky Gut Syndrome."

Normally the openings in the G.I. mucosa are less than three microns. However, these opening, which should admit to the body only very tiny particles of food are now able to admit large particles, greater than 5,000 daltons in size, of undigested food.

Normally the large molecules of food would not be absorbed but be carried out of the body and down the toilet. Not only are large molecules of incompletely digested food introduced into our bodies but so are large toxic substances.

Once these large holes are created, more and more different foods may enter the body. Through antigen-antibody reactions, the body doesn't recognize these molecules as "friendly food," but as foreign bodies. This is because of the size of the food molecules. Instead of the person reacting to one food, they now react to many. A vicious cascade of events is occurring. I have treated people who have so many food allergies that, out of the 96 foods that are traditionally tested, they were only able to consume a dozen with immunity.

❦ SYMPTOMS OF FOOD ALLERGIES

The following psychological and physical symptoms are some of the indicators of food allergies:

Psychological Symptoms
Anxiety, aggressive behavior, inability to concentrate, confusion, crying spells, excessive daydreaming, inability to make decisions, depression, chronic fatigue, poor work habits, indifference, irritability, learning disabilities, mental dullness, mental lethargy, panic attacks, personality changes, and restlessness.

Physical Symptoms
NERVOUS SYSTEM, GENERAL: Dizziness, chronic fatigue, excessive drowsiness, faintness, hyperactivity, hunger with binge or spree eating, insomnia, sleepiness soon after eating, slurred speech, stuttering, restless leg syndrome, and weakness

HEAD: Feeling of fullness in the head, headache

EYES, EARS, NOSE, AND THROAT: Runny nose, stuffy nose, excessive mucous formation, watery eyes, blurring of vision, ringing in the ears, hearing loss, recurrent ear infections, itching ears, ear drainage, sore throat, chronic cough, excessive gagging, canker sores, itching of the roof of the mouth, recurrent sinusitis, and hoarseness

HEART AND LUNGS: Palpitations, increased heart rate (tachycardia), asthma, congestion in the chest

GASTROINTESTINAL: Nausea, vomiting, diarrhea, constipation, bloating after meals, belching, colitis, flatulence (passing gas), feeling of fullness in the stomach long after finishing a meal, abdominal pains or cramps (The medical term commonly used to describe these symptoms is Irritable Bowel Syndrome.)

SKIN: Hives, rashes, eczema, dermatitis, pallor, dark circles under the eyes (shiners)

MUSCULAR-SKELETAL: Muscle aches and pains, joint aches and pains, swelling of the hands, feet, or ankles, lack of muscular control

GENITAL AND URINARY TRACT: Urinary frequency, urgency, vaginal discharge, discharge from penis

🌺 CAUSES OF FOOD ALLERGIES

Obviously many foods can cause allergies. However, the most common ones are wheat, corn, citrus, chocolate, eggs, dairy products, shellfish, peanuts, and yeast. Not surprisingly, these are the foods most frequently found in our diet.

It has been shown that people can even be allergic to water, so imagine what possibilities there are. I am sure there is not a food in existence that some poor soul is not allergic to.

🌺 TESTING FOR ALLERGIES

The immune system is composed of two armies of defense. As mentioned earlier, these are the B and T cells. First is the humoral system, made up of B cells, and the second is the cellular system, consisting of T cells. The T cells, secreted by the thymus gland, form leukocytes and lymphocytes that are cells that circulate through the body, seeking and engulfing infectious foreign germs and particles. They also help B cells.

The B cells form proteins. One of these proteins, as discussed previously, is IgE and it is used by the antibodies that counteract the allergic substance or allergen.

Several methods of testing may be used to determine the cause of allergies.

Skin Test

An allergic extract is introduced under the skin and, if the person is allergic to the substance, within fifteen to twenty minutes a welt rises, reddens, and enlarges. This test is not very accurate for chemical and food allergies.

There are two skin tests: scratch and intradermal. In the first, the skin is broken by scratching with a needle, introducing the extract into the body. In the latter, an extract is introduced through a needle just under the surface of the skin.

Measurement of Total IgE in the Bloodstream

A person who is highly allergic has an elevated level of this protein.

R.A.S.T.

The patient's blood is drawn and tested in the laboratory for specific allergic substances, such as chemicals, pollens, molds, danders, and foods.

Cytotoxic

This is a new test with some limitations in that the patient's blood is taken and tested. It is primarily restricted to food allergies.

Sublingual Testing

Several drops of the potentially allergic substance are placed under the tongue and the patient is observed for a reaction. This test is very time-consuming but, depending on the observer, is quite accurate.

Kinesiology

In this test the operator checks the strength of body muscles while exposing the patient to specific foods. Weakness of the muscles indicates a positive allergic reaction to the food.

E.A.V. Instrument (Electroacupuncture)

There are numerous testing instruments in this category. In general, a probe is placed on the allergy meridians of the patient's fingers and toes and tested for weakness in the energetic patterns when specific foods are placed in the circuits. I have found these instruments to be safe, accurate, and inexpensive to use. However, the cost of purchasing these instruments is high and they require specialized training for their operation.

Subjection Avoidance

The food or other suspected substance is introduce the food or other substance to the person and observe the individual's reaction. It is similar to sublingual testing. In this case, a diary is kept by the patient. For example, one would record the time the food was ingested and the time and kind of reaction that occurred, if any, as well as the severity of the reaction. The diary should be kept for a minimum of one week, but, ideally it should be kept for three weeks.

In avoidance treatment, the allergic substance is withdrawn from the person's environment, but usually for three weeks and, again, the patient keeps a diary to determine whether the symptoms previously experienced, disappear.

☙ APPROACHES TO TREATMENT OF ALLERGIES

The treatment of allergies is broken down into four approaches:
- The avoidance of the allergic substance.
- The use of medications in removing the symptoms.
- Strengthening the immune system so that the body is able to defend itself from the assault of the allergic substance. Remember, treatment involves the total reassessment of one's life-style.
- In the case of food, the use of specific substances that counteract the action of an individual food that you are allergic to.

Avoidance practices improve symptoms by decreasing the exposure to the allergic substance. It is important to proceed with an avoidance system as soon as one finds the source of the allergy. This may be essential and even lifesaving, particularly in cases in which the immune system is weakened and overwhelmed. In extreme cases, it may be necessary to live a Spartan life-style. In other cases it is simply not possible to avoid the allergen.

❦ Frequently Seen Contact, Inhalant, or Airborne Allergens

- Cat hair: Slippers, toys, cheaper furs
- Dog hair: Rugs, cheaper furs, and robes
- Horse dander and hair: Automobile seats, pillows, blankets, mattresses, stuffing, carpet pads, furniture, clothes lining, wigs, bags, glove s, hats, and furs.
- Rabbit hair: Angora sweaters, collars, scarves, dyed furs, fur-lined gloves, dresses, felt hats, toys, lapin fur. Many times rabbit is sold as chinchilla, sable, fox, or seal.
- Goat hair: Doll hair, wigs, upholstered furniture, bedding, brushes, mohair covers, suits, linings.
- Fur: Made from mink, rabbit, goat, skunk, and muskrat, they are important causes of hay fever. The dyes from the furs may cause dermatitis. Many furs are sold under different names.

ACTUAL FUR	LABELED AS
Mink, dyed	Sable
Muskrat, dyed	Mink, sable, seal
Otter	Sable
Goat	Bear, leopard
Opossum	Beaver
Rabbit	Sable, fox, seal, chinchilla, ermine

- Feathers and Animal Dander: Most frequently seen are from horses, cows, chickens, geese, ducks, pigeons, parrots, canaries, rabbits, guinea pigs, cats, and dogs.
- Feathers: The feathers from the birds mentioned above, plus turkeys, along with feathers of other household BIRDS or PETS are found in furniture, pillows, feather beds, comforters, dusters, dress and coat trimmings, and hats.
- Sheep Wool: This may also cause symptoms and it can be found in mattresses, furniture, clothes, blankets, toys, and car seat covers.

❧ Avoidance Regimens for Airborne Allergens

Avoidance regimens improve symptoms by decreasing exposure to allergens that trigger the allergic reaction. Avoidance may completely relieve allergy to foods, drugs, and animals. However, because seasonal pollens and molds typically have widespread airborne distribution, complete avoidance is difficult, if not impossible. Steps that can be taken to reduce exposure during the pollinating seasons include:

- Limit outdoor activities such as hikes or drives through the country.
- Remain inside in an air-conditioned environment.
- Wear a face mask when exposure is likely to be greatest.
- Temporarily move to a pollen-free environment.

To reduce perennial allergen exposure in the home, efforts should be made to create at least one allergen-free room where the patient can spend most of his time. Reduction of the allergen load for part of the day can help decrease symptoms significantly. The following are suggestions for reducing exposure to common household allergens:

Dust

- Enclose mattresses, box springs, and pillows in vinyl or synthetic coverings. Be careful if small children will be using these.
- Eliminate upholstered furniture, stuffed toys, carpeting, wall hangings, and other dust collectors from the room.
- If possible, use hardwood, vinyl, or tile floors, and painted, paneled, or wallpapered walls. Avoid products with toxic fumes.
- Wet mop and vacuum frequently; a water-filtered vacuum system may be useful.
- Maintain clean, adequate filters for home heating and air-conditioning systems to avoid disseminating of allergens throughout the house. Special filtering systems are available.

Molds

- Use dehumidifiers, fungicidal sprays, and mold-resistant paint in damp, moist areas including basements, laundry rooms, bathrooms, and storage areas.

- Eliminate dense vegetation around the house.
- Avoid raking leaves and other activities involving decaying vegetation; use a face mask when this exposure cannot be avoided.

Danders
- Eliminate pets from the home. If household pets are indispensable, keep them outside to reduce distribution of danders in the home.
- Face masks may be useful for sensitive people with occupational exposure to animals.

Other
- Eliminate nonspecific irritants from the home. These include smoke, vapors from cleaning fluids, or other odors that may trigger nonspecific mast cell reactivity and symptoms.

Regarding food allergies, avoidance may completely relieve the symptoms. However, this, too, is not always simple because there is such an extensive alteration of food by commercial food producers. Chemicals are sprayed on the soil or on the plants and fed to the animals. In addition, chemical food additives are examples of only one of many unnatural substances that are used, and many of these products may produce allergies. This list is infinite and includes preservatives, dyes, weed killers, steroids, and antibiotics, to mention a few.

❧ THE PERILS OF ICE CREAM

In the good old days, when ice cream was made with whole eggs, milk, and sugar and laboriously cranked in the old home freezer, a serving of ice cream was an occasional family treat and did not cause much harm.

However, today, in this mass-production, synthetic age, there is a very good possibility that you are treating your family to another poison if you buy some supermarket products.

Ice cream manufacturers are not required by law to use natural products in their products. Consequently, the majority of ice creams are synthetic from start to finish. Laboratory analyses of some ice creams have shown the following ingredients:

- Diethyl glycol – a cheap chemical that is used as an emulsifier instead of eggs. It is identical to the chemical used in antifreeze and in paint removers.
- Piperonal – used as a substitute for vanilla. This is a chemical used to kill lice.
- Aldehyde C17 – used to flavor cherry ice cream. It is an inflammable chemical that is used in the manufacture of aniline dyes, plastic, and rubber.
- Ethyl acetate – used to give ice cream a pineapple flavor. It is also used as a cleaner for leather and textiles, and its vapors have been known to cause chronic lung, liver, and heart damage.
- Butyraldehyde – used in nut-flavored ice cream. It is one of the more common ingredients of rubber cement.
- Amyl acetate – used for its banana flavor. It is nitrate solvent.

The next time you are tempted by a luscious-looking sundae or banana split or ice cream soda, KNOW the source of the ingredients. Otherwise you might be ordering a mixture of antifreeze, oil, paint remover, nitrate solvent, leather cleaner, and lice killer and you may not find it quite so appetizing.

❄ Food Additives

To date our government allows more than 4,000 additives to be put in our foods.

While one must read the labels on packaged foods, some ingredients are not included as they are protected by the government as a "secret recipe" of the manufacturer. Therefore, the label could say it may contain either one substance or another and by not telling you which is actually used in the product, the true ingredients are not revealed.

❄ Treatment for Food Allergies and Reactions to Additives

Avoidance System
My recommended avoidance program is called a diversified rotary diet and works as follows:

After testing and identifying the foods that you are allergic to, you must totally avoid these foods for a two-month period. During this time you may eat the foods that you are not allergic to but you must not eat them more than once every four days.

After two months, you may introduce one of the foods to which you are allergic. WARNING: Introduce only one food at a time and after the first time, do not try it again for one week. It is usual that about 5 percent of the foods the patient originally reacted to may never be tolerated; however, other foods may ultimately be eaten without symptoms.

Use of Medication

There are many medications on the market but they fall into just a few categories. First are antihistamines. Their function is to block the action of the histamine that does the damage in allergies. Unfortunately, most antihistamines have the side effect of causing drowsiness.

Second are the decongestants that decrease congestion, as the name implies. Unfortunately, they tend to stimulate the person and cause an increase in heart rate along with a rise in blood pressure.

Next is the steroid class of drugs that includes cortisone; with their prolonged use many side effects may be produced, some quite serious.

People who have severe allergic reactions to food or insects should carry the drug adrenaline with them so they can inject themselves as needed to prevent an acute allergic reaction.

Desensitization shots are sometimes used. In this case, small amounts of the reacting allergen is injected, stimulating the body to defend itself.

The antigen is diluted so no serious reactions occur but an immunity is created. To continue the immunity, the shots need to be given periodically, very commonly once a week.

You may get similar results by placing drops of the allergen under the tongue where it is rapidly absorbed into the body. When the exact dilution is found, it does not cause an allergic reaction but normalizes the person's response to the antigen. We have a good treatment when symptoms go away.

This works well for foods. In the case of sublingual treatments, when a patient is allergic to a specific food, if you take a tiny bit of that food before consuming a quantity of it, it is possible that you will be protected and consequently not experience an allergic reaction. Another therapy is colostrum, which is found in mother's milk during the first several weeks after birth. As the newborn suckles, he or she gains newly created antibodies. These antibodies protect the newborn from infections that are found naturally in the environment. This is important because the newborn's immune system is usually not fully matured and functioning at maximum capacity. The milk of the cow gives similar responses when administered to adult humans.

Colostrum is marketed by a number of nutritional companies. The dose is usually one teaspoon twice daily if you are suffering from flu or cold. As a preventive, one teaspoon daily. In children, ½ teaspoon daily for chronic allergy patients as well as the treatment of cold and flu.

When these antibodies are isolated and given to an individual who has allergies, if the immune system is in good function, the person will not have an allergic reaction.

A relatively new therapy is enzyme-potentiated desensitization (EPD). This is a method of immunotherapy developed by Dr. Leonard M. McEwan in England in the 1960s.

In this process, desensitization of the reacting allergens occurs. The patient is administered extremely diluted doses of these allergens with an enzyme called B-glucuronidase. This enzyme potentiates the resistance to the allergen at the cellular level, hence prolonging the body's response for up to three months. All of the allergic products, including foods, chemicals, food additives such as formaldehyde, detergents, petrochemicals, pollens, molds, and insect bites, are utilized.

The conditions that may be treated are extensive, and include almost any in which the immune system is involved. They include hay fever, rhinitis, asthma, hives, eczema from foods and food additives and preservatives, multiple chemical sensitivities, Attention Deficit Hyperactivity Disorder (ADHD), Autism, Irritable Bowel Syndrome, Krohn's Disease, ulcerative colitis, migraines, rheumatoid arthritis, ankylosing spondylitis, and system lupus. This represents a partial list of problems that EPD therapy improves. The treatment is given every three months for a minimum of six treatments.

Most people respond favorably to this treatment. In some cases there has been a reported 90 percent favorable response. This therapy has been used in many other countries since the 1970s. In fact in England, the government has banned traditional allergy shots except when administered in a hospital. They are not allowed in a doctor's office because of the possibility of life-threatening reactions. EPD, because of its safety, is the only therapy given in the physician's office. This therapy is now being offered in the United States to a limited degree.

In my medical practice, I have observed phenomenal results with EPD. One patient who was very allergic to molds and dust was literally forced to remain in bed for days during a severe allergic attack, which commonly afflicted her on windy days. After I administered EPD treatments her life returned to normal and she rarely experienced a reaction to allergens.

Homeopathic Remedies

One of the most effective ways of treating allergies, whether to airborne or food substances, is with homeopathic remedies. Many of these products block the action of specific substances. By way of combining with the offending allergens, homeopathic remedies can render them harmless. In this case, instead of suppressing the symptoms, they actually neutralize the substance. These are safe and without side effects, whether injected under the skin or intermuscularly(into a muscle), inhaled, or taken sublingually. These remedies are able to rapidly relieve the symptoms.

Strengthening the Immune System

The last and probably one of the most effective approaches to the treatment of allergies is to strengthen the immune system. It is a realistic approach that strengthens and builds a healthy body in order to counteract any attack from outside and will be one of the most effective treatments for the future.

The first technique has existed for some time and is called "immunotherapy." This is a treatment in which a small amount of the allergy-producing agent is collected and injected into the individual in increasing amounts over a period of time. This eventually neutralizes the antigen, or attacking substance.

To strengthen the immune system naturally, one must apply the same general principles used in any health-promoting program. The triad for this program is adequate exercise, positive attitude, and good nutrition. These three areas are very effective and easy to implement.

First, one should exercise daily or at least every other day. One should work the cardiovascular system for a minimum of 20 minutes. If there is a special medical problem, such as hypertension or heart disease, the exercise should be performed only under a physician's guidance.

One objective of the human body is to move and exercise in order to stimulate the circulatory system to do its job—to nourish the muscles and carry off waste. Other substances, such as endorphins, are released during exercise. Endorphins promote healing and establish a feeling of well being in the body.

Thoughts are very powerful in promoting health. Negative or fearful thoughts actually interfere with the body's normal functioning. (See Chapter 4 for more.) One technique is to visualize the antibodies attacking the allergic agent and quickly consuming or carrying off the particles without creating any harm to the body.

Nutrition plays an immense role in a healthy immune system. The consumption of sugar and other refined carbohydrates reduces the speed with which the white blood cells destroy and attack substances within the body. This effect lasts up to four hours. One soft drink reduces the speed of removing a foreign substance, therefore allowing it to remain in the body longer to cause damage.

Increase your intake of dietary fibers; soluble and insoluble fibers that come from Jerusalem artichokes, oat and wheat bran, carrots, and peas. These products not only detoxify the intestines but also stimulate the growth of friendly bacteria such as lactobacillus acidophilus and bifidobacteria bifidus. These friendly bacteria promote proper digestion of foods and also activate enzymes and vitamins. They also release beneficial short-chain fatty acids, which nourish the intestinal mucosal, thereby assisting in repair and the production of new cells.

Also add to your diet additional supplementation of acidophilus and bifidus for the same reasons. Because only so many living organisms can occupy the same space, if you have a large population of friendly bacteria, that leaves less space and a food supply for the pathogenic bacteria.

Avoid the foods that commonly cause allergies. For example, peanuts could be a problem. A mold, anti-flavin, is often found growing on peanuts and many people are sensitive to this mold.

In general, a good diet, free of sweets and refined carbohydrates, should be the goal.

Vitamin and mineral supplements are essential to good immune system functioning. There are four elements that protect our system against foreign bodies. They are vitamins A, C, E, and the trace element, selenium, which are mentioned in Chapter 4. My expression is, "ACES protect us."

Initially, when a person is overwhelmed with the allergy, three days of intravenous buffered vitamin C brings great relief. The dosage should be high; about 45,000 to 60,000 milligrams daily. This method bypasses the digestive tract so the body can receive the benefit of all of the vitamin C. Normally, only 50 percent of ingested vitamin C is utilized.

Another vitamin is pantothenic acid, B5, that works with the adrenal system whose function is to protect the body against stress and external attack. One must again take higher doses than recommended under the RDAs; up to 2000 milligrams daily.

Zinc helps the thymus gland to function. Since our defending cells are produced by the thymus, zinc will help. Research shows that zinc lozenges, taken every two hours during the day, can reduce the length and severity of common throat viruses and some allergies. In the case of a severe allergic reaction, 50 milligrams of zinc taken hourly during waking hours definitely reduces the allergic reaction. It is a very powerful antiallergic substance.

Amino acids are important as well. For instance, the amino acid Arginine should be given daily. Its function is to stimulate the immune response by enhancing the production of T cells. However, one must avoid high doses in cases of schizophrenic conditions. Also, one should not take high doses of a single amino acid for a prolonged period; rather a balanced formula is indicated.

Next, since many food allergens are from a protein base, and many of them are absorbed in a largely undigested condition that our systems cannot handle, we need help to further break down these proteins. This is done by a digestive substance called hydrochloric acid (HCL). Therefore, giving additional HCL with each meal helps to break down the protein molecules into smaller, easily handled substances. Be sure that you do not have a gastrointestinal ulcer condition before you begin this therapy.

Lastly, cleansing the system is important. Fasts are very effective to cleanse the body of accumulated toxins. A three-day diet of fresh apples and pure water is a good way to do this. (See Appendix A.)

🦋 ALLERGIC CHILDREN

Children have special problems of allergies and the immune system. Many babies who are the offspring of allergic parents suffer from early allergic problems. They begin having colicky spells, abdominal cramping, and gas. They also experience frequent diaper rash and eczema. One reason is that they are given too many foods too quickly. Foods such as eggs, orange juice, and red meats generally should not be introduced until after six months or, if possible, even later, at eight months of age. This is because the digestive tract of the child may be poorly developed and if exposed to many foods, the child will not be able to fully digest them. They may then become allergic to these foods very early. As the allergic child grows up, he may begin to experience repeated infections of the ears, nose, and throat. The results of the recurrent infections are a hearing problem due to repeated accumulation of fluid in the ears (serous otitis media); and adenoiditis, causing a chronic nasal discharge and a nasal type speech. Other symptoms are recurrent fevers and loss of appetite. There may also be respiratory problems such as wheezing and coughing. This pattern may cause many problems for the child, interfering with his normal activities even to the extent of keeping him away from school. He may also have a tendency to have warts, which could be a sign of decreased immunity.

A specific example is that of a child by the name of Michael, who

I saw in my practice. Michael was four years old. His mother brought him into my office in a panic. She had just been told by an ear, nose, and throat specialist that if her son didn't have tubes placed in his ears he could become deaf. The history was typical. As a baby, Michael was colicky. Many foods that he consumed created problems for him. He had gas, bloating, cramping, diarrhea, irritability, and crying. After he reached his first birthday some of these symptoms lessened, but were replaced by other symptoms. He began to have recurrent sore throats and ear infections. Actually, at least every two months, he would complain of painful ears and of being hard of hearing. His mother took him to physicians that always prescribed antibiotics. The infection eventually improved, only to reoccur soon.

This pattern went on for several years with the infections seemingly getting worse and more frequent. Even the occasional swimming pool adventure had to be eliminated, as the outcome was always the same — a bad ear infection occurred.

Now we come to the crisis; serious consequences if something isn't done. An examination revealed the typical reddened, swollen ear drums and canals slightly shiny and bulging from pressure from the middle ear. Also, there were edematous tonsils. Remember, the tonsils function as a lymphatic filtering system, trapping and destroying bacteria and allergens in the mouth and throat region. Michael's mother stated that another physician did suggest that it might be necessary to remove the tonsils as well. The effect of allergies caused an infectious state to become established. Challenging the integrity of the tonsils and mucosal lining of the nose took its toll.

After a review of the case, including Michael's early history, I made several recommendations:

First, I administered a homeopathic shot to strengthen his immunity. (In this case I chose Nigersan.) Second, I administered homeopathic drops into the ear for ten days. Third, I immediately started Michael on a program of vitamins and minerals, including 3,000 mg. of vitamin C orally per day; 25 mg. of zinc daily (initially in the form of zinc lozenges, after a week reduced to 10 mg. daily). Lastly, I recommended an immediate change in his diet. He was to avoid all dairy, sugar, citrus, eggs, and wheat for two months, and substitute rice or soy milk for cow's milk and rice or soy bread for other grain breads. After two months on this program, he was to be evaluated to see if any of the restricted foods could be integrated into the diet.

In additional, because of Michael's problems caused by recurrent antibiotic therapy, I suspected Michael was suffering from an intestinal yeast overgrowth. I began him on acidophilus therapy to re-establish his normal bowel flora. There was probably some damage to the bowel lining as well.

I re-examined Michael after one week, again in one month and again one month later. I found the infection totally gone and the ears looked normal. I continued to see Michael periodically over the next two years. During this period, he had no evidence of an ear infection or hearing loss. In addition, his tonsils, which had been reddened and swollen, were now normal in size and looked healthy. This allowed his normal lymphatic system to remain intact and on the job. Little by little, I was able to introduce some of the prohibited foods back into Michael's diet. However, for some time I kept him away from dairy products to which he was obviously very allergic.

This is an example of what allergies can cause. When recognized and properly treated, a profound change in a child's life can result. Actually, I have examined and treated over 100 similar cases and in each case I have seen a significant improvement in the child's health.

❧ OTHER THINGS WE CAN DO

The treatment of this condition in children is similar to that of adults. It is necessary to evaluate the child's environment, particularly considering household pets and the type of pillow he uses. It should be made of a synthetic material rather than feathers. Curtains should be replaced with Venetian blinds to reduce dust collection.

Most important is the child's diet. In my practice, I have observed children who have had two to three years of recurrent sore throats and ear infections improve dramatically after milk and other dairy products were eliminated from their diet. Of course, a product such as soy milk should be substituted in its place. It would also be valuable to remove sugar, citrus, and wheat from the diet. It appears that reducing the total load of allergens, food and airborne, helps the immune system heal. This often leads to further dramatic improvements.

Since these children need calcium as it may be blocked from absorption by allergies, I would recommend extra calcium at bedtime. This also has the ability to relax them and help them sleep. I would also recommend a maintenance of extra chewable or crystalline vitamin C. This may result in a general increase in the health of the child who now has the ability to fight off allergic, viral, and bacterial insults to the body. If the child is beginning to come down with a cold, give him or her chewable zinc lozenges every two hours during the day to completely prevent the cold or at least cause the infection to be very mild and shorten the time of the disease.

I found that one very important aspect of respiratory problems, such as asthma, is the emotional status of the person. The allergic child who lives in a highly stressful environment where there is conflict in the family and where he receives excessive criticism may be unable to assert or express himself, holding in his feelings. Those feelings may result in being unable to completely expand the lungs, causing the lack of good air exchange. This causes the child to struggle for air and, because of bronchial spasms, the child does not receive enough air.

Breathing exercises work well as a therapy because it encourages forced lung expansion. The exercise also distracts the child from the emotional problems.

These simple steps may totally change the life of a child. Parents have said that they have seen a very dramatic difference in the behavior of the child including his being more content. School performance may also improve.

It is important to start working with this health challenge at an early age to diminish the possibility that the allergic child will grow up to be an allergic adult.

These health rules generally apply to an adult as well. One should take the appropriate steps to treat the allergy and achieve good health.

REFERENCES

Crook, William G., M.D. *Tracking Down Hidden Food Allergy*. Jackson, TN: Professional Books, 1980.

_____. *You & Allergy*. Jackson, TN: Professional Books, 1980.

Tierney, Lawrence M., Jr., M.D., Stephen J. McPhee, M.D., Maxine A. Papadakis, M.D., Steven A. Schroeder, M.D. *Current Medical Diagnosis & Treatment*. Norwalk, CT: Appleton & Lange, 1993.

🌿 FOOD RESPONSE ASSESSMENT

How do we know that we are allergic to certain foods? Here is a program that will help you evaluate foods for potential allergies.

How to Prepare Foods
Choose 21 foods that you suspect you might be allergic to. Next choose one of these foods to test. Steam vegetables to tender-crisp, or eat raw. Soak grains or beans overnight, then cook on low-heat until ready. Bake, steam, or boil potatoes. Soft boil or poach eggs. Broil or bake meat, fish, or poultry.

Prepare Yourself Mentally
Before you test this first food, sit, relax, and put your total positive attention on what you are doing. Record your pulse rate on the Food Response Diary along with the time you start eating each food. Record the food, if it is raw or cooked, and your general feelings when you start eating. Make a mental note or set a timer to record your responses to the eaten food after a half hour, one hour, an-hour-and-a-half, and two hours.

Monitor Your Body
Before eating, during eating, and after eating, be mindful of your general feelings and specific areas of your body, such as eyes, ears, nose, mouth, heart, skin, joints, head, etc. Now eat the food, by itself, slowly, and stay aware of your chewing, the texture of the food, the taste, and the smell.

Meaning of Responses or Lack of Responses
If you feel well during the two-hour test period and your pulse does not lower or raise more than 8 to 10 beats per minute, you have an acceptable food for your customized Response Food Plan.

If you respond by any degree of severity in any of the response ways, your body cells are signaling that this food is not for you at this time.

What Are the Usual Signal Responses?
If your body's cells definitely respond in one or more of the following ways at the half-hour intervals, record these signs in your Food Response Diary. Stay mindful of emotions.

ABDOMEN
Belching
Bloating
Cramps
Diarrhea
Hyperacidity
Nausea
Rumblings
Thirst
Vomiting

MUSCLES
Ache
Jerk
Spasms
Weakness

SKIN
Cold/Clammy
Flush
Ghostly
Heat
Hives
Itch
Perspiring

EARS
Aching
Blocked
Hearing loss
Itching
Ringing
Sensitivity to sound

HEART/LUNGS
Chest Pain
Cough
Pressure
Rapid Breathing
Rapid Pulse
Starved for Air

HEAD
Migraine
Mild headache
Pressure
Throbbing

GENERAL FEELINGS
Chilly/cold
Crying
Dizzy
Faint
Fatigue
Heaviness
Hot Flashes
Stimulated
Tense

PERCEPTION
Disorientation
Dream-like
Hallucination
Insomnia
Paranoid (persistent)
Wandering

THROAT/MOUTH
Acid Taste
Bad Taste
Hoarse
Itch (frequent)
Sore Throat
Sore Tongue
Teeth Hurt
Tender Gums
Tight Throat

JOINTS
Ache
Heat
Sharp Pain
Stiffening
Swelling

SPEECH
Reading errors
Sluggish
Stammer

MOODS/ EMOTIONS
Anxious
Fearsome
Hyperactive
Intoxicated
Irritable
Listless
Negativity
Talkative

FOOD RESPONSE ASSESSMENT
Food Response Diary

TIME	FOOD, DRINK, MEDICATION	TIME	SYMPTOMS & FEELINGS

CHAPTER II

Multiple Sclerosis: New Hope

DESCRIPTION OF MULTIPLE SCLEROSIS

MULTIPLE SCLEROSIS, or MS, is a chronic and slowly progressive neurological disease that predominantly strikes young adults living in the temperate zones. It appears that people living in the tropical zones are not at risk for this disease. However, people of European ancestry are at higher risk. Diagnosis can usually be made by a cranial MRI, a thorough history, and a physical examination.

The characteristic pathology of MS is the destruction of the myelin sheaths that insulate nerve, brain, and spinal cord fibers. Symptoms include numbness and tingling of the extremities, double vision, loss of equilibrium, urinary problems, and muscle weakness.

The disease goes from rapid progression of symptoms to minimal symptoms of the disease or remission. It becomes then a cyclic disease as symptoms may disappear for days or weeks and then reappear. Symptoms may be triggered by stressful emotional situations or environmental events, such as excessive heat or chemical exposure. As more and more of the nervous system is destroyed, the patient may eventually be confined to a wheelchair or even become bedridden.

Although cortisone, given in high doses, may help for a short time, there is currently no cure noted in medical books.

Some recent studies reveal that a new drug called interferon beta-1b has some effect on slowing down the progress of multiple sclerosis. (IFNB Multiple Sclerosis Study Group, April, 1993) Also, over the last several years, research done by Dr. Hans Nieper of Germany shows promise in retarding the disease process safely. (Nieper, Hans, MD, November, 1992). The hypothesis is that calcium EAP (ethanolaminophosphoric acid) (INNB Multiple Sclerosis Study Group, April, 1993), which is calcium linked to an amino acid, can easily be taken up by the nerve tissues. This appears to protect and repair the myelin sheaths. Calcium EAP, which is manufactured in Germany but is now available in the U.S., is given both orally and intravenously.

For people living in the tropics, where the sun shines longer producing strong ultraviolet rays, calcium is laid down more effectively by the production of Vitamin D. This may explain why multiple sclerosis is practically unknown in the tropics.

罂 HOMEOPATHIC SOLUTION

Another treatment is the use of homeopathic medications that heal any infection in the vicinity of the nervous system. There may also be a major autoimmune component of multiple sclerosis that involves substances such as microbes or complex proteins. These products may cause a localized inflammatory reaction within the nervous system causing a self-destruction process. The key is that certain homeopathic remedies are able to block this damaging reaction. Another beneficial effect of homeopathic remedies is that they cause the immune system to, on its own, internally produce interferon, a substance that combats disease.

Another key to the overall treatment is detoxifying and cleansing the body. Purging the intestinal tract with herbs removes toxins from the body. (See also Appendix A.) Eating organically grown, healthy foods, which are free of chemicals, is preferred. Animal products should be used in moderation, thereby reducing large amounts of complex proteins, which react in the body. Vegetable protein is much more easily digested and assimilated by the human system.

Nutritional therapies that are also beneficial are supplementation with vitamin C, 4-8 grams daily; beta carotene, 20,000 units daily, Dynogenol, 100 mg daily, and multiminerals, both macro- and micro-nutrients.

A very important part of the cleansing program is exemplified by a study done in England recently. A British physician treated over 2,100 patients with multiple sclerosis. He used only two procedures. First, he had all of the amalgam fillings removed from his patients' teeth and replaced them with porcelain compound. Next he gave them dietary supplements consisting of high levels of vitamins and minerals, particularly vitamin C. Of this group of patients, approximately 1,200, or more than half, improved substantially.

It is not 100 percent proven how the silver fillings affected the multiple sclerosis, unless it was a result of the mercury used in the production of the silver amalgam. It is well known that mercury has a great affinity for nerve cells and causes substantial damage to the brain and peripheral nerves. It is also well known that in some people mercury causes other disorders.

Aromatherapy

A very effective modality used successfully in the treatment of MS is application of aromatherapy. First diffuse the essential oils citrus, ylang ylang, tanacetum, patchouly, and lavender. This combination can be diffused in a blender. (This should be done as discussed in Chapter 7.) The time is one hour in the morning and one hour at either noon or in the evening.

In addition, massage the following formula of essential oils on the neck, spine, and feet:

sandlewood	4 drops
peppermint	2 drops
geranium	12 drops
juniper	6 drops

Combined with the cleansing of the body and the injection of nutritional supplements, the essential oil program is very effective in improving MS.

Physical therapy is also an essential part of the program. This helps lessen the muscle spasticity and keeps the muscles mobile and strong. Needless to say, a good positive attitude is very important, as well as a flexible thought pattern.

I have observed patients go into remission with this program. Their strength and balance improve and they feel a new sense of freedom and hope.

REFERENCES:

Henry, John Bernard, MD. *Clinical Diagnosis & Management by Laboratory Methods*. Philadelphia: W.B. Saunders Company, 1991.

Enby, Erik, MD, Peter Gosch, and Michael Sheehan. *Hidden Killers: The Revolutionary Medical Discoveries of Professor Guenther Enderlein*. Sheehan Communications, 1990.

IFNB Multiple Sclerosis Study Group. "Interferon beta-1b is effective in relapsing-remitting multiple sclerosis. I. Clinical results of a multicenter, randomized, double-blind, placebo-controlled trial." *Neurology*, April 1993.

_____. "Interferon beta-1b is effective in relapsing-remitting multiple sclerosis. II. MRI analysis results of a multicenter, randomized, double-blind, placebo-controlled trial." *Neurology*, April 1993.

Kobler, Franz MD. *Calcium EAP*. Dr Franz Kobler Chemie GmbH, Germany.

Nieper, Hans MD. "Review of Non-Toxic Therapy." *Journal of the International Academy of Preventive Medicine*, Vol. 7, No. 3, P. 5-10, Nov. 1982.

Tierne, Lawrence M., Jr., M.D., Stephen J. McPhee, M.D., Maxine A. Papadakis, M.D., Steven A. Schroeder, M.D. *Current Medical Diagnosis & Treatment*. Norwalk, CT: Appleton & Lange, 1993.

CHAPTER 12

A Healthy Approach to Diabetes Mellitus

A VERY SERIOUS DISEASE

IT IS ESTIMATED that six million people in the United States suffer from diabetes, an endocrine malfunction leading to high blood sugar. This condition is caused when either the pancreas doesn't produce enough absolute insulin or the insulin that it produces is ineffective.

Diabetes sufferers fall into two categories: people who generally require the addition of insulin from an external source (Type I Diabetes); and those who do not need insulin (Type II Diabetes). The latter type usually responds well to a diet management program, with or without oral medication to control the level of blood sugar.

The diagnosis of diabetes is made through a family history, as there is a tendency for it to be hereditary; by a history of symptoms such as excessive thirst, hunger, and urination; and by measuring laboratory values of high blood and urine sugar.

Human organs are somewhat protected from damage against elevated blood sugar. However, there are three exceptions to this—the nerves, the eyes, and the kidneys.

In cases of prolonged diabetes serious damage may occur to these organs. Peripheral neuropathy is the result of damage to the nerves resulting in numbness of the extremities. (I once treated a woman with insulin dependent diabetes who had stepped on a thumbtack 24 hours earlier and hadn't felt a thing. I discovered this because the tack was still in her foot when I examined her.) Blindness is seen in some advanced diabetes cases. Kidney damage can be so severe that renal failure is sometimes observed and kidney implant is occasionally indicated.

The more chronically advanced disease causes many other problems such as accelerated atherosclerosis, ulcers and gangrene in the extremities, loss of balance, impotence, nausea and vomiting, and even in extreme conditions, coma and death. It is obvious from these complications that this is a very serious disease.

🦋 THE HOLISTIC SOLUTION

How do we treat this disease holistically? There are eight major features within the treatment:

1. Diet
2. Medication — Allopathic
3. Medication — natural
4. Intravenous chemical intervention
5. Nutritional Supplements
6. Exercise
7. Behavioral counseling
8. Meditation

Diet

Is diet important? Absolutely! Often the proper diet can prevent a mild diabetes from converting into the more serious type of diabetes creating the need for daily insulin shots or perhaps oral medication.

To further describe the effects diet has on this disease, I present a published study and personal observations. Our Native American population has a very high incidence of Type I *Diabetes Mellitus*. How did this happen? The following hypothesis was presented. Due to the western Native American populations' history of being hunters and nomads, they moved with the buffalo and antelope herds. When they had abundant game, they ate well. However, there were times when there was no readily available food. Although they didn't have the convenience of refrigeration, they made jerky in order to preserve the meat. Consequently, they experienced days with little intake of food, hence few calories. During these times they needed to have substantial blood sugar levels in the body in order to create the energy to continue life and go hunting for more meat.

The theory goes that certain groups of Native Americans genetically and naturally developed a gene that produced prolonged, elevated blood sugar and, most importantly, allowed them to survive in times of temporary food deprivation. (To understand this you need to know that the liver has the ability to store a readily available form of sugar used for energy.) Additionally, they had another regulating life-style feature — exercise. Because they normally were very active physically their blood sugar was brought down to normal; in other words, they burned up the sugar through physical exercise. Also, they were able to maintain their normal weight. This is important as it has been shown that excessive fat cells block the body's normal response to insulin.

The problems began when our Native American population changed their life-style. Most have moved from their comfortable houses with open hearths for cooking. Also they have left behind their gardens out back, which offered a ready supply of fresh vegetables and grains, and they exercised while they cared for and harvested the garden. They have replaced these gardens with modern food stores and the foods high in refined carbohydrates, fats, and salt that are available there. These foods tend to overload the metabolism as well as the circulatory system and produce atherosclerosis and obesity.

Yet, even though many Native Americans completely changed their diet and exercise regimen, they still carry the gene that causes sustained elevation of blood sugar.

To see an overweight Native American is common now, just as it is among much of the rest of the U.S. population. However, photographs taken of these proud Native Americans around the turn of this century show that an overweight person was rare.

One must recognize that the present diet, along with a lack of exercise, may produce a full-blown case of diabetes with all of its complications. It is believed that although the body has a tendency to manifest diabetes if the genetic predisposition is present, we can slow down or even prevent the whole process by changing our lifestyle, especially through diet management and exercise.

DIETARY RULES: HOW DO WE TREAT THIS PROBLEM?

First, complex carbohydrates, which are slowly absorbed and therefore do not stress the pancreas, should make up 45 to 50 percent of the diet. Furthermore, most of the carbohydrates should come from fruits, vegetables, seeds, grains, and legumes, and as much of the diet as possible should be eaten raw or only lightly cooked. The other 50 to 55 percent should be split between fat and protein. One should include lots of fiber that again slows down the absorption of carbohydrates and fats and dilutes the intestinal tract.

A good example of an ideal food for diabetics is Jerusalem artichokes, sometimes called sun chokes commercially. These contain an insulin sugar. This sugar is metabolized and assimilated by the liver rather than the pancreas and is an excellent source of energy for diabetics. If possible, those with diabetes should consume Jerusalem artichokes daily.

Another area in the diet to be aware of is food allergies. Apparently, if you are allergic to some foods, a reaction is set up that causes excessive stress on the pancreas. Consequently, one should make an effort to identify any allergic foods and eliminate them from the diet.

Certain foods, such as fruit juices, and in particular orange juice, are largely simple sugar and cause an elevation in blood sugar just as any other sweet would. It is important to restrict these foods.

It is also important to repair a damaged bowel that has a defective filtering system and may admit large amounts of sugar to the blood stream. Vitamins A and C are important in the repair process, as is the beneficial bacteria Acidophilus.

It is also important when you eat. Since most digestive, as well as physical, activities go on during the day, it is important to consume a good, balanced breakfast and lunch, but a very light evening meal. Caloriewise, 80 percent of your nutrition should be consumed before 2:00 P.M.

Medication — Allopathic

Medications are indicated in some situations. In milder cases, oral hypoglycemic drugs are successful. The chemical name for these is sulfonylureas. When taken before meals, they are helpful in lowering the blood sugar.

In more serious cases, insulin injections are required to control blood sugar. In these cases the insulin must be administered one or more times daily, without fail. In cases in which the pancreas is not producing any significant amount of insulin, the patient's life depends upon careful administration of this drug.

If the balance of this treatment program is followed carefully, then it is reasonable to expect that the need for the hypoglycemic drugs as well as insulin may be reduced. According to my clinical experience, in some cases they may even be eliminated completely.

Medication — Natural

One of the more innovative natural approaches to treating diabetes is "Live Cell Therapy, " which is based on the theory that cells from an active animal organ may support or stimulate the function of the human organs. Even in the case of poorly functioning organs we may see beneficial results.

The pancreas of an unborn calf or sheep is extracted surgically. The animal extract is purified so that it is safe and pure, and it is given orally or intravenously or intramuscularly to the diabetic. The diabetic's pancreas usually begins to operate on an improved level. The therapy is continued twice a week for a month. Thereafter it is administered monthly until maximum function of the pancreas occurs (usually within several months). I have found that 50 percent of the patients receive a benefit from this therapy. Some are able to reduce their insulin doses.

Another therapy from which my patients have benefited dramatically, specifically in the cases of peripheral neuropathy, is homeopathic medications. In particular, an intravenous injection of Mucokehl, a homeopathic product formulated and distributed by Sanum Company of Germany, is capable of rapidly opening up circulation, consequently improving blood flow in the small arteries and capillaries. In the case of diabetes the sensations of the extremities return to normal and blood flow improves. Mucokehl also repairs damaged peripheral nerves.

One of my patients who was an insulin dependent for 20 years called me an hour after his first shot of Mucokehl, claiming that the feeling in his feet and legs, which was nonexistent prior to the therapy, was now 45 percent of normal. Ongoing therapy, including four more shots each a week apart, resulted in the sensation in his lower extremities becoming 80 percent normal.

I have found this homeopathic treatment to be effective in many cases with similar complications. This is particularly significant if you take into account that the medical literature suggests that the condition of peripheral neuropathy can never be reversed. No diabetic with nerve or circulatory injury should be without homeopathic therapy.

Intravenous Chemical Intervention
Chelation, as described in Chapter 9, is used to open up the vessels of the lower extremities and kidneys so that the blood flow is improved. Often I have observed that after a few chelation treatments kidneys that were in mild failure opened up and began filtering normally. These treatments also improve peripheral tissue circulation. This is a treatment that should certainly be tried.

Nutritional Supplements
Of course, balanced nutritional supplementation is essential, particularly the antioxidant vitamins and minerals A, C, E, and the trace element selenium (ACES).

Other products also appear to help, including the mineral chromium. According to reports, chromium assists sugar metabolism at the cellular level. Moreover, a study of juvenile diabetics revealed that they suffered from an absolute reduction of total body chromium levels. Therefore, there is a need for extra chromium with juvenile diabetes.

According to reports, another helpful mineral is vanadyl sulfate, which is derived from the metal vanadium. Early studies show that this mineral may naturally lower blood sugars. Reports from French literature around the turn of the century reveal that this mineral helped diabetics. My experience in using this mineral in the treatment of diabetes has been very encouraging. More study should be done on vanadyl sulfate, though in the meantime it is safe to take.

Note however that chromium and vanadyl sulfate should not be used together as they may be antagonistic to each other.

Exercise

Sugar is a source of energy that allows muscles to create movement. Therefore, regular and consistent exercise is essential in the control of diabetes. Another effect of exercise is that it helps to reduce weight and improves circulation.

Again exercise, insulin, and other medications, taken as a unit, should be carefully monitored. Be certain that the blood sugar level does not drop abruptly. At times it may be necessary to reduce the amount of insulin and other medications when exercising.

Behavior Counseling

It is very important that the diabetic maintains regularity, consistency, and moderation in their lives. If the patient develops a good and consistent schedule then blood sugar levels are more easily manageable. They should attempt to rise and take their medication at the same time daily. They should eat approximately the same amount of calories at the same time each day. They should exercise daily. They should control stress as much as possible as this also affects the blood sugar level.

In all cases the blood sugar level should be carefully monitored by your doctor or with a home blood sugar analyzing unit. Also, if there should be any significant change in exercise, diet, stress, even lack of sleep, then adjustments should be made in the medication.

Lastly, according to some studies, diabetics have certain personality tendencies. In some but not all cases, diabetics have a tendency to excesses in their lives. Again, moderation is the keyword when dealing with diabetes.

Since the abrupt elevation or the reduction in serum sugar levels can have potentially disastrous consequences, I cannot emphasize enough that any changes in therapy must be carefully monitored by your primary care physician. I feel that in some cases, self care may be hazardous. The therapies mentioned here are indeed powerful!

CHAPTER 13

Are We Parasitized?

NONRECOGNIZED DISEASE

IN 1965 I WAS FORTUNATE to study for some time at the National Institute of Tropical Disease in Mexico City. There I became aware of the immensity of the problem of parasites in the human body.

One investigation done by Mexican Public Health at that time involved examination of the contents of the stools of cooks and dishwashers at restaurants frequently patronized by American tourists while in Mexico City. This study revealed that the stools contained multiple parasitic infestations. Considering the poor sanitation in Mexico, this was not surprising.

In 1964 I served for a time as a medical missionary in the mountains north of Mexico City. I experienced parasitism first hand and found that this problem ran rampant because of the poor living conditions that continue to exist today. These unfortunate people use water that is not treated, and they all drink from a common well or stream. At the time I was there I even watched a 26-year-old man die of complications of amoebic abscess of the liver.

❧ A Major World Problem

Microbial parasites kill more people around the world than AIDS and cancer combined. According to a study published in American Health magazine in March 1992, parasites with their consequent complications are the number two killer in the world. Parasites such as ascaris lumbricoides alone infect unknown millions of persons annually and are said to be responsible for the deaths of 20,000 people each year. Schistosomiasis, transmitted by infected water and causing vomiting of blood and grossly enlarged spleens and livers, severely affects 20 million victims in Africa, Asia, and South America.

Filariasis causes elephant-shaped limbs and enlarged testicles. The World Health Organization claims that more than two million new cases are reported annually in India and elsewhere in the world.

Malaria is responsible for killing more than one million people a year and infects some 300 million others.

All of these are examples of parasitic conditions. In general the number of persons being infected by parasites annually is grossly on the increase, quadrupling in the last fifteen years.

Another interesting fact about parasites is that new species are still being discovered. For instance, cyclospora outbreaks have been reported recently. A protozoa travels on fruits, it was not known by experts four years ago and only recently was included in medical texts.

❧ The United States Has a Problem as Well

In the United States parasites cause a variety of problems. Hookworms tend to cause anemia or deficiency in blood that, if severe enough, may result in fatigue, poor appetite, and even in advanced cases, shortness of breath. The common mode of entrance into the body is by way of the feet when one is walking barefoot in the dirt.

In April of 1993, the city of Milwaukee, Wisconsin, experienced an acute gastrointestinal infection, when thousands of residents drank improperly treated city water. A parasite, cryptosporidia, was isolated both in the water and in the intestinal tracts of the afflicted, linking the cause and the effect. Those afflicted suffered from symptoms that included fever, vomiting, diarrhea, and flulike problems, such as aches and pains of the muscles and joints. While some people had self-limiting symptoms (which means they went away on their own after a time), many of those afflicted had to be hospitalized in order to stabilize their fluid losses and other symptoms.

🐛 A Can of Worms

Another parasite, ascaris lumbricoides, or roundworm, can enter the body when the person eats vegetables that are contaminated. Remember that many of our vegetables and fruits are imported from Mexico where sanitation is not up to the standards of our own country. This parasite not only can cause bowel upsets but also, in many cases, ends up in our lungs and upper respiratory systems—noses and sinuses. There are reported cases of this parasite producing asthmatic symptoms. I feel that all patients suffering from upper respiratory problems should be routinely investigated for roundworm.

Many children with chronic stomach aches may have giardiasis of the intestines. This is an annoying problem causing abdominal pain, intestinal spasm, and occasionally nausea.

🐛 Protozoas

More serious are the findings of chronic diarrhea in children who live in unsanitary environments and contact amebiasis, a type of protozoa. This parasite may cause ulceration of the intestinal lining, along with bleeding. Worst of all it may go undetected because of the difficulty of isolating the parasite or because the family physician may not think of it as a diagnosis. It could ultimately lead to dehydration, anemia, and even death.

Some parasites, such as filariasis, clog the lymphatic system and cause poor circulation as well as increased risk of infection from other diseases.

Skin rashes may be a result of parasites invading the outside or dermal layers and ultimately penetrating deeper and going through their entire life cycle while residing in various organs.

While other parasites may not have such a profound effect on our health, they may still cause such problems as upset stomach, or gas and bloating, while others are known to cause both constipation and diarrhea. This last symptom may lead to dehydration, shock, and even hospitalization if the diarrhea is severe enough. Nevertheless, even if parasites cause mild symptoms, they should all be identified and eliminated from our bodies. They can stress our immune system, deplete our nutritional resources, create an environment for other infections, and generally interfere with our overall good health and well-being.

❦ OTHER SIMILAR PROBLEMS

According to statistics, 70 percent of "traveler's diarrhea" is caused by bacteria and viruses. In contrast to a parasite that may take days to produce symptoms, these infections cause symptoms usually within hours of ingestion. While the symptoms may be severe, the infections could be self limiting, so the symptoms may not last too long. When treated, usually with antibiotics, the time of infection is shortened. If not treated, as a rule, symptoms disappear in several days to two weeks without leaving serious residual effects. (An exception to this is typhoid, produced by the germ Salmonella. In this case you are acutely ill and you generally have a fever and diarrhea.) This situation is in sharp contrast to parasites, which may persist for months and even years if untreated.

❦ WHAT IS THE PROBLEM OF DIAGNOSIS?

In 1970, after returning from Mexico to the United States to practice, I observed the numbers of immigrants who recently arrived from foreign countries. I was certain that many of these individuals were suffering from intestinal parasites. After all, the Customs and Immigration Department does not routinely check for this problem.

However, trying to confirm this was quite difficult, at times requiring that as many as eight or nine stool specimens be sent for laboratory testing before a positive sample was found. My queries to pathologists as to why the tests were so inaccurate were met with both indifference and denial. I found that most pathologists were not personally examining the specimens but were delegating the responsibility to technicians, who were less familiar with parasites. Furthermore, during processing of the specimen material, the parasite was often altered by fixatives and preservatives and the time delay between collection and examination was frequently prolonged. Often the eggs and larva were destroyed by these processes and, therefore, could never be identified.

🥀 WE IGNORE THE PROBLEM

The cavalier attitudes of the primary physicians were either that the parasites stopped at our borders or that their presence created no problem here. They ignored that valuable nutrients were being robbed from us by these creatures, not to mention that damage was being done to the intestinal mucosa and other tissues and that general allergic reactions were being caused in many cases.

Because of my frustration with the situation, I located a pathologist who specialized in parasitology. I found his test results to be very accurate.

🥀 CAN WE ADAPT?

After a period of time the body seems to have an adaptive mechanism. An example is that if you ingest the eggs or the actual parasite, within a few days they multiply and cause an irritation to the stomach and bowel lining. Then the symptoms, including fever, aches and pains, vomiting, and diarrhea, last days and sometimes months and even years.

These symptoms happen for a reason. Primarily irritation and damage to the gastrointestinal lining speed up its activity and movement. This actually benefits the individual because both vomiting and diarrhea accelerate the dumping of the bowel and stomach and consequently reduces the overall population of the parasite within our body. While this is one of our protective mechanisms, it could become detrimental if too much fluid and electrolytes or salts are lost. We then suffer from dehydration and electrolyte imbalance. This could be dangerous and even fatal, particularly for small children and infants because they have less fluid reserves and can't always communicate to us their need for these extra fluids.

After the acute phase, which usually lasts for several days (but the period of time is variable), two things happen. Either because of treatment or because of the person's own natural immunity, the parasite is totally eliminated. Or, and this occurs frequently, a period of stabilization happens in which the patient still has the parasite but the serious symptoms disappear.

At this point the person technically becomes a "carrier," though he or she is often totally unaware of his or her condition. Nevertheless, although the more profound symptoms no longer exist, he or she may still exhibit mild or subtle symptoms, such as fatigue, bloating, mild abdominal discomfort, dyspepsia, poor digestion, and poorly formed stools. One may notice small amounts of blood or mucus in the stool or a fair amount of undigested food coming through the system. Even a frequent sense of nausea or an easily upset stomach may be present. These insidious symptoms don't have to occur daily, but may occur once a month or even less often.

While the symptoms are minor they do persist, sometimes for years, as the person accepts this condition as normal for themselves. Nevertheless, problems are occurring inside. At times there is chronic damage to the bowel mucosa. Small amounts of bleeding may occur, which over time translates into significant blood loss anemia.

✾ Autoimmune Reaction

Also the damage to the mucosa may disrupt the natural bowel filtering system, thus allowing abnormal products to enter the body. Large chain proteins may be admitted to the blood stream that could cause autoimmune or other allergic reactions.

✾ Why Are They Called Parasites?

Another big issue between the body and parasites is their competition for food. Some parasites require similar nutrients as the human body and consequently may rob us of adequate nutrition. Don't forget that parasites mainly live in the intestinal tract and therefore have the first opportunity to approach our food supply. Other parasites feed on bacteria and may reduce the total amount of our natural bowel flora.

Remember that beneficial bacteria such as acidophilus help us to digest our food so that it is more easily assimilated. This symbiosis (living together with a benefit to both life forms) relationship may be disrupted. The result could be dysbiosis (living together but causing harm to one or the other life form).

❦ An Unfriendly Agent among Us

Of course another obvious problem with a person who is a carrier of a parasite is that while they are not being treated, they pose a threat to people around them. If they fail to wash their hands after going to the bathroom, the parasite eggs and the parasite itself may be found on their hands and under their fingernails. Consequently if they are involved in food handling then the organism may be transferred to food and unknowingly ingested by the next victim of parasitosis.

Not surprisingly, due to the mobility of the population and the number of households containing pets, also a ready source of parasites, I have found that nearly 15 percent of my patients possess parasites or pathological bacteria of some kind in their guts. What is more important is that there is an improvement in energy and general health when my patients are treated for parasites. I often see a healing of some chronically resistant disease states after these parasites have been satisfactorily treated and eliminated.

❦ A True Life Example

Eleanor was raised during the era when one didn't question one's omnipotent doctor. (Come to think of it, we are still largely in that era, aren't we.) As did most women of her generation, she had spent much of her 74 years ingesting various prescription drugs and medicines, including diet pills, sleeping pills, pep pills, tranquilizers, diuretics, antihistamines, barbiturates, amphetamines, pain killers, and a multitude of antibiotics. In fact, at the time of this particular incident, Eleanor had seven different unidentified pills in her pill dispenser and over 30 bottles of various prescriptions in the medicine cabinet.

In the spring Eleanor became ill and after several days of nausea, gas, stomach pain, and burning on urination, she went to see her new doctor for the first time. After a urine analysis and office visit, he determined that she had a "bladder infection" and he prescribed an antibiotic. After several days, the antibiotic hadn't cured the problem, so Eleanor returned to the doctor. He prescribed a different antibiotic. This one caused Eleanor's eyes to swell and itch, but did not cure her "bladder infection." At yet another visit her doctor prescribed a different antibiotic. This time Eleanor broke out in hives. Another visit, another antibiotic; this one appeared to have some beneficial effect, without serious side-effects, so she continued to take it.

At the beginning of May Eleanor and her sister left for a ten-day cruise to the Caribbean, a trip they had planned for nearly a year. By this time Eleanor had been taking antibiotics almost continuously for two months. During the cruise she became extremely ill with nausea, stomach aches, vomiting, and diarrhea. The ship's doctor gave her a shot of an unknown medication and she spent the last four days of the trip in bed. During this time she was unable to hold down most food or liquid.

The symptoms continued after Eleanor returned home. She returned to her doctor who, after an examination, pronounced that she had the "urinary infection" again and prescribed another antibiotic. However, the symptoms persisted and Eleanor had trouble keeping any food — even water — down. She began losing weight, and she reached the point where she could barely get out of bed. After she called him, the doctor prescribed another antibiotic and antinausea medication. Eleanor's symptoms worsened. A few days later, after another phone call to a doctor filling in for her "out-of-office" doctor, she was provided with another antibiotic prescription and one for antinausea suppositories. However, the symptoms continued to worsen.

After a few more days of sheer misery, her primary doctor recommended that Eleanor see a gastroenterologist. The specialist scheduled Eleanor for a complete series of tests that required 12 days to accomplish. These tests, all requiring laxatives, enemas, and dyes, included running scopes up, down, and all around as well as X-rays, MRIs, and ultrasounds. The only thing found was a small polyp in Eleanor's colon. The specialist was convinced that while the polyp should be removed in the near future, it was not the cause of her severe nausea, vomiting, and stomach pain. His only suggestion was to rerun all of the tests in case something had been missed.

By this time, six weeks after the boat cruise, Eleanor was completely bedridden, had lost 31 pounds, and was existing entirely on sips of water every 15 minutes and broth—and, of course, her antibiotics, diuretics, estrogen, and other pills. She was becoming severely dehydrated and weak. After she consulted with the gastroenterologist, he agreed to admit her to the hospital. There they ran more tests, with more laxatives, enemas, and dyes, and more scopes up, down, and all around, and they still found nothing new. More specialists were called in and more tests were run.

At this point the doctors conferred and decided that Eleanor must have cancer of the pancreas! The family was called in and told the catastrophic news; pancreatic cancer is nearly always fatal. The doctors admitted their diagnosis was essentially a "rule out" one, that they had decided that Eleanor had pancreatic cancer because they just couldn't find anything else wrong, They scheduled Eleanor for exploratory surgery.

Eleanor's surgery was performed on Saturday morning, ten days after she had first been admitted to the hospital. The surgeon opened her up abdominally and examined her pancreas—and found NO CANCER!!! However, while the surgeons were in the abdomen they removed the section of the colon that had the polyp. Fortunately, IT WAS NOT MALIGNANT!!!

However Eleanor's story is far from over. The source of the original problem had not yet been found! The day after the surgery, the doctors conferred again and decided that as soon as Eleanor had recovered sufficiently from the surgery, all of the tests would be rerun. This would require more laxatives, enemas and dyes, more scopes up, down, and around, more X-rays, MRIs and ultrasounds.

Meanwhile, for the first five days after the surgery, Eleanor proceeded to heal "normally." However she still could not eat or drink anything without experiencing nausea, vomiting, or stomach pain. By this time she had been in the hospital for 14 days and had essentially nothing to eat or drink but small sips of ice and a continuous intravenous solution of water and electrolytes with 5 percent sugar. (It is interesting to note that when Eleanor finally was served a meal after having nothing but water for nearly 10 weeks, she was given a roast beef sandwich—very hard to digest.)

After 17 days in the hospital, Eleanor was discharged.

To summarize, up to this point Eleanor:

1. had been on several different antibiotics for an extended period of time. These antibiotics had been prescribed by doctors who had spent a total of maybe 10 minutes examining her and by other doctors who had not even seen her.
2. had gotten very sick on a vacation cruise.
3. had had a complete gastrointestinal work-up.
4. had been pronounced as having "fatal pancreatic cancer."
5. had had major surgery that only proved that she did not have cancer.
6. had had a portion of her bowel removed.
7. spent 17 days in the hospital with nothing to eat or drink except "sugar water" administered intravenously.
8. had lost 32 pounds.
9. still had the original ailment!!!

Fortunately, this is not the end of Eleanor's story!

The best thing to happen to Eleanor since this saga began was to get her out of the hospital. She was still having severe stomach pains, could not keep most food down, and was so weak that she was bedridden. It took her major effort to go to the bathroom. By this time, for all practical purposes, Eleanor had not been out of bed for over 11 weeks. However, she did manage to occasionally keep down some high-calorie, high-protein, high-vitamin food supplement liquids. In the meantime the family searched for alternate treatment. They contacted me through the Arizona Homeopathic Medical Association. Because of the era in which Eleanor was raised, she was at first reluctant to consider alternative methods. However, at her families' insistence and due to her recent experiences with traditional medicine and reassured by the fact that I am an M.D., she hesitantly agreed to see me.

Her first visit with me was a complete shock to Eleanor and her family. I spent over two-and-a-half hours listening, asking questions, reviewing her past records, and taking pages of notes. By the end of the interview, I knew Eleanor, her complete medical history, and a very large portion of the entire family's. I then made two definitive statements:

1. Eleanor was depleted of most nourishment. We needed to immediately get her started on a series of health-rebuilding intravenous treatments containing megadoses of vitamins, minerals, and amino acids.

2. I was relatively certain that she had contracted a parasite on her Caribbean cruise that had completely devastated her digestive system.

I started the intravenous treatments that day and scheduled an appointment with the parasitic diagnostic lab, one of the few in the western U.S. capable of testing for these diseases.

The lab test results confirmed that Eleanor had major parasite infestations in her intestinal tract. She also had a yeast infection in the intestinal tract. Both of these could have been minor problems, but due to the destruction of Eleanor's natural intestinal defense system by all of the antibiotics, both diseases flourished and had became major problems. In fact, in conjunction with the dehydration, they very nearly led to her demise!

I prescribed a medicine to eliminate the parasites and a homeopathic medicine for the yeast infection. I also told her to immediately stop taking antacids (which she had been using by the handful) and instead to take hydrochloric acid (the opposite of antacid) in order to aid digestion. I also added acidophilus, orally, to her diet to replace her bowel flora.

We gave Eleanor a number of intravenous therapies during the next two weeks. The ingredients included electrolytes, sugars, amino acids, and vitamins, with particularly high doses of vitamin C.

Within days Eleanor displayed considerable physical improvement and a major attitude adjustment. She began taking larger amounts of liquids and quickly progressed to solid food, which she was able to hold down just fine. She also completely changed her life-style.

She began eating "healthy"—fresh fruit, raw vegetables, chicken and fish while eliminating beef, pork, cheeses, milk, and sugar. She also began taking vitamins and minerals and drinking herb teas and rice milk. Within a couple of weeks, her appetite returned and she was eating regular meals without nausea and stomach pain and without taking handfuls of antacid tablets.

On September 5 (less than two months after being diagnosed as having fatal pancreatic cancer), Eleanor renewed her driver's license and began, for the first time since April, doing some shopping on her own. In early October she began doing volunteer office work for the Easter Seal Society! By November, she went on salary, full time—at 74 years of age!

⚘ The Proper Approach

The correct approach to the problem of parasites is obviously to first have a proper diagnosis. If a person has symptoms of acute stomach bloating, excess gas expulsion, mild abdominal discomfort, and chronic or acute diarrhea, nausea, or vomiting, consider the diagnosis of parasites, particularly if the diagnosis has not been previously made. This is especially true if you have traveled out of the country where sanitation is not up to our standards. Even if you were only in a foreign country for a day, this diagnosis should still be considered. Remember only one meal or glass of liquid can cause an infection.

Furthermore, seek out a physician who is knowledgeable about parasites. Always inquire as to his or her experience.

Next insist upon a laboratory that specializes in or certainly has had much experience in identifying parasites. Also make certain your stool specimen isn't being held for days prior to the examination as the parasite might have disintegrated and become undetectable.

If the first specimen is negative, make certain that follow-up specimens are collected; even the best laboratories miss from 20 to 60 percent of the parasites on the first analysis. It may take up to eight specimens before the parasite is finally found. Remember these are living organisms and they possess a defense system that allows them to survive. The parasites literally have the ability to hide, very often avoiding proper detection.

Once the diagnosis is made, be assured that the proper treatment is utilized. Each parasite requires a different therapy because there are different types of species, Some are one-celled, some are multi-celled, and some are much more complex.

Lastly after the therapy has been completed, recheck the stool to see if the parasite is truly gone. Even if you feel better, all that you may have done is weakened the parasite temporarily or reduced its population. It could multiply and become a threat to you once again.

In conclusion, I recommend that in all cases where parasites are suspected, the physician be persuaded to persist in trying to locate the little critters.

✺ PREVENTION — THE KEY

As with any disease, prevention is the key to good health. So what can you do to protect yourself against parasites?

A Healthy Life-Style

First, strive for a healthy life-style. Eat well — pure food and water. Exercise regularly. Take vitamin supplements, particularly vitamins A, C, and E. Vitamin A protects and repairs your mucosa, particularly in the respiratory and digestive tracts. Vitamin C improves the immune system. Vitamin E improves your circulatory system. Include mineral supplements in your program.

Next prepare your food well. If you are not totally convinced of the pure source of your vegetables, then wash them thoroughly and soak them in water with a few drops of iodine or chlorine (household bleach will do) for at least 12 minutes. If there is any question about the purity of the water, then boil it for five minutes before drinking it. Remember, night soil (that is, human waste) is often used as fertilizer in foreign countries. We here in the United States receive much of our fruits and vegetables from other countries.

Be aware! Parasites can survive in ice. Therefore, even if you drink bottled products, if you drink them over ice you could get sick.

In the case of meats, cook them well. Heat, if applied long enough, kills parasites and their larva (the immature phase of the adult) and destroys the eggs. Raw beef and pork are often sources of tapeworms and trichinosis. Raw fish also harbors many parasites. An example is a Fluke infection that could be life threatening.

Traveling to Foreign Countries

Anyone who travels outside the U.S.A., particularly in areas that have less than good sanitary conditions, should suspect parasitic infection if they have chronic gastrointestinal problems. Parasitism and "travelers diarrhea" are common, and these tips may save your life.

First, know your source of food. Always ask questions. Some hotels are more cautious than others and have purified water, for example. As a rule, drink bottled water or other bottled drinks without ice.

Be very careful of fresh vegetables, particularly salads and fruits, even though they look great. The old adage "looks may be deceiving" is especially true here, as these bugs are so small that they cannot be seen with the naked eye.

❧ TREATMENT

As mentioned earlier, remember that all parasites are not the same, so treatments for them must be different. There are a number of medications—products containing citrus extract and artemisia, for example. These are considered to be natural products. Regarding commercial products, mebendazole and oxantel parnoate are used for roundworm. One exceptionally fine new drug for the treatment of both amebiasis and giardiasis is tinidazole. While this product is not available in the United States, it is marketed under the name of Fasigyn in Mexico. It is given in the amount of 2 grams, one time only, and has no serious side effects. Also for these parasites, Yodoxin, an iodine-based product, has remarkable curative effects.

Preventive Medication

As a preventive, I recommend several products. First, for those persons who don't have a stomach ulcer or gastritis, you may benefit from hydrochloric acid, marketed under the name of Betaine Hydrochloride. This can be ingested with each meal. Taking it ensures that you have a plenty of acid in your stomach, which is important because many times acid will destroy the parasite and its eggs in the stomach, before it reaches your intestinal tract and gets firmly established there. So take hydrochloric acid daily.

Second, taking one teaspoon of Bentonite every morning coats the intestinal tract and prevents the parasite from grabbing the mucosa and establishing itself. It also kills certain parasites. Bentonite is a chalky material found in most health food stores and some pharmacies. It is safe to humans.

Next, use an oral bulking agent, such as oat bran, apple pectin, psyllium seed powder, or rice bran, daily. Bulking agents mechanically eliminate the parasites and their cysts and eggs by way of brushing and in some cases binding up these organisms.

Use garlic extensively! It is a natural antibiotic and destroys the bacteria that many parasites need to survive.

🦠 If You Have Parasites

If you go abroad, take along some Lomotil. This product stops severe diarrhea, prevents dehydration, and allows you to maintain your travel schedule.

If, when you have dysentery, an intravenous solution of vitamins, minerals, and sugar is not readily available, drink products that contain electrolytes and sugar. There are numerous products on the market. An example is bottled fruit juices diluted with an equal amounts of water. They must be diluted because, in the case of dysentery, you lose a proportionally higher amount of liquids than with other products. Therefore when using commercial products you should generally dilute them with water.

In an urgent situation with children, I have found that coke syrup is a very successful, simple treatment. You can obtain coke syrup at a soda fountain. Children need the sugar in the coke for energy, but carbonation causes more gas. If coke syrup is not available, then boil coke for five minutes in an open pan, then let mixture cool. Small children usually like the taste of this remedy, which is important as they normally have no desire for food when suffering from dysentery. This is one of the few times in my practice that I recommend a soft drink.

The other product is acidophilus, which establishes your normal bowel flora and brings your gastrointestinal tract back into balance rapidly.

Your diet is also important. If you are certain about the cleanliness of cabbage, eat it raw. When eaten raw, it sweeps the bowel tract clean. If fact, it is said that one leaf of cabbage can kill and remove one million worms.

REFERENCES

Collins, Chic. "Mom's Misadventures with the Malevolent Medical Monster," Phoenix, Arizona, 1992.

Gittleman, Ann Louise. *Guess What Came to Dinner: Parasites and Your Health.* Garden City Park, NY: Avery Publishing Group Inc., 1993.

Kanagel, Robert. "Boot Camp for Parasitologists." From *Science Illustrated,* January/February, 1989, Vol. 2, Number 6.

Tierne, Lawrence M., Jr., M.D., Stephen J. McPhee, M.D., Maxine A. Papadakis, M.D., Steven A. Schroeder, M.D. *Current Medical Diagnosis & Treatment.* Norwalk, CT: Appleton & Lange, 1993.

CHAPTER 14

Yeast and Its Effects on Our Health

THERE'S A FUNGUS AMONG US

SYMPTOMS SUCH AS FATIGUE, depression, headaches, lack of ability to concentrate, skin rashes, dyspepsia (gas, bloating, and pain), diarrhea or constipation, respiratory difficulties (coughing, wheezing, phlegm), hearing problems, nasal congestion, and hyperactivity may indicate an infection caused by the fungus Candida albicans. This is a living organism that is commonly called yeast and normally lives in the human body beginning shortly after birth.

Different kinds of yeasts, such as brewer's and baker's yeasts, exist in everyday life. Other types are found in the fermentation processes of beer and wine. Although yeast organisms are normally found in the body to some degree or another, they may flare up at certain times and increase in numbers. It becomes a serious problem when yeast grows abundantly and spreads uncontrolled throughout the body.

Various factors cause the flare-ups. Among them are: excessive stress; antibiotic therapy; a diet loaded with sweets, alcohol, and refined breads; damp or humid weather; ingestion of certain drugs (particularly birth control pills and prednisone); and other accompanying diseases and viruses such as Chronic Fatigue Syndrome.

Because of the abundance of these conditions, candidiasis, or yeast infection, is seen quite frequently in medical practice. Yeast infection may not be easily recognized, however, since it mimics other diseases with similar symptoms. For instance, chronic or recurrent sinusitis as well as postnasal discharge may be caused by excessive yeast. One patient who experienced a nasal discharge for 12 years was cured in 24 hours when I applied an antifungicide to her nasal area. Also, recurrent ear infections involving both the middle and outer ear may be caused by fungus and are sometimes contracted from a swimming pool. Frequent bladder infections may involve a yeast component. Indigestion, gas, and bloating can be caused by excessive yeast growth, as well.

Many skin rashes are related to fungal infections. These may also be seen under the finger- and toenails, causing a white or yellow discoloration and leading to the loss of one or more nails. At times the organism may be carried by the blood stream to other organs of the body and interfere with their proper functioning as well.

PMS, or premenstrual syndrome, marked by abdominal cramps, headaches, and weakness, is a serious problem from which many women suffer. This illness is found to be associated with candida infection in many cases. If the yeast infection is cured and B_6 and magnesium are given as supplements, I have seen many PMS cases clear up completely. Vaginal infections are commonly caused by candida albicans, especially when they are recurrent or when antibiotic therapy has been used prior to the infection.

Another important aspect is that candida albicans secretes substances, called neurotoxins, that, when released naturally or after their destruction, may cause neurological problems as well as memory loss. This process can also depress the immune system so the patient is more susceptible to other infections.

How are these organisms identified? Laboratories may detect the organism by a swab that is cultured. Also a blood test can be performed to detect their presence. A good history is helpful in identifying the organism.

✺ TREATING YEAST INFECTIONS

Once a diagnosis is completed, proper treatment is imperative. A good diet, one that is high in protein and complex carbohydrates, is the most important aspect. It is particularly important to avoid all types of sugars (simple carbohydrates), yeast-containing foods including bread, fruit juices and dried fruits, dairy products, vinegar, alcohol, pickles, and any foods that are fermented.

Specific treatments of a vaginal infection caused by yeast include glycothymolin, one of the most effective and safest therapies. The treatment is to douche with one teaspoon per quart of water daily for ten days.

Other important aspects of therapy for intestinal and systemic yeast include taking digestive aids, such as both betaine hydrochloric and bile salts. Also take multivitamins, with emphasis on vitamin A with betacarotene, vitamins C and E, minerals, particularly zinc, essential fatty acids including evening primrose oil, biotin, immune supporters like vitamin B, thymus glandular tissue, and taheebo tea, sometimes marketed under the name of "Pau d'Arco tea." Include herbs and homeopathic remedies, especially garlic, in your therapies as well. Homeopathic extracts of candida are very effective in destroying the organism. Remember, acidophilus should always be taken to restore normal bowel flora when you have completed the treatment of Candidiasis.

Other pharmaceuticals are also available and include Nystatin, Nizoral, and DiFlucan. Unfortunately, these medications have side effects that may also be hazardous, particularly to the liver.

A special ultraviolet lamp has been found to be safe and effective in treating the candida fungus. One or two treatments may be all that is required. The C brand ultraviolet lamp is pulsed at specific frequencies and placed approximately six inches from the skin at the site of infection. If the fungus infection is internal, the lamp is placed six inches from the blood vessels under the tongue while the mouth is open. This area is rich with superficial blood vessels and is a site for the administration of many sublingual medication such as nitroglycerin used in heart conditions. At this site absorption is rapid and complete.

In all of these therapies be cautious not to move too aggressively as one could experience headaches, agitation, or fatigue—the effects of rapid "die off." This is a phenomenon observed when the organism is killed off too quickly and the products of waste from their internal structure, such as neurotoxins, accumulate.

Also very important are other improvements in life-style, such as getting plenty of exercise, sunshine, and rest.

At the end of this chapter appears the Canditrak History/Symptom Worksheet, a questionnaire used by doctors to determine if a patient has a problem with yeast infection.

REFERENCES:

"Canditrak History/Symptom Worksheet." Norman, OK: CeroDex Laboratories, Inc., 1985.

Crook, William G., MD. *The Yeast Connection: A Medical Breakthrough*. Jackson, TN: Professional Books, 1986.

Tierne, Lawrence M., Jr., M.D., Stephen J. McPhee, M.D., Maxine A. Papadakis, M.D., Steven A. Schroeder, M.D. *Current Medical Diagnosis & Treatment*. Norwalk, CT: Appleton & Lange, 1993.

SURVEY OF POTENTIAL YEAST INFECTION

To determine if you may have a yeast infection, answer the following questions. If you answer "yes" to:

1. Two or more of the "History" questions, you could have a yeast infection;
2. Six or more of the "History" questions, the likelihood that you will get a yeast infection is quite high;
3. Ten or more of the "Symptoms," you have a probability of having a yeast infection; or
4. Twenty or more "Symptoms" and three or more "History" questions, you have a high probability of having a yeast infection.

HISTORY – Have you:	Yes	No
1. taken antibiotics frequently?	____	____
2. taken antibiotics for a long period of time (30 - 60 days).	____	____
3. taken Prednisone or other steroids?	____	____
4. taken a product called Flagyl?	____	____
5. been repeatedly exposed to pesticides, fertilizers, or other chemicals?	____	____
6. been diagnosed as having parasites?	____	____
7. had a long history of allergies?	____	____
8. Do you notice your symptoms after exposure to damp or humid days or when residing around lakes?	____	____
9. Do damp and humid areas bother you?	____	____
10. Do you crave sugar?	____	____
11. Do you have chronic fungal infections such as athletes foot, jock itch, recurrent ear infections?	____	____
12. Does tobacco smoke bother you?	____	____
13. At times, has the consumption of sugar made you feel as if you are drunk?	____	____

SURVEY OF POTENTIAL YEAST INFECTION

Symptoms of Yeast Infection	Yes	No
1. Lethargy?	_____	_____
2. Fatigue?	_____	_____
3. Irritability?	_____	_____
4. Inability to concentrate?	_____	_____
5. Poor memory?	_____	_____
6. Sleepiness?	_____	_____
7. Feel out of touch with surroundings?	_____	_____
8. Headache?	_____	_____
9. Blurry vision?	_____	_____
10. Recurrent ear infections?	_____	_____
11. Muscle weakness?	_____	_____
12. Dry or sore throat?	_____	_____
13. White coating on tongue/inside of mouth?	_____	_____
14. Persistent skin rash?	_____	_____
15. Persistent nasal discharge?	_____	_____
16. Wheezing?	_____	_____
17. Heart palpitations?	_____	_____
18. Persistent constipation?	_____	_____
19. Persistent diarrhea?	_____	_____
20. Gain weight easily?	_____	_____
21. Bloating?	_____	_____
22. Indigestion?	_____	_____
23. Belching?	_____	_____
24. Pass gas frequently?	_____	_____
25. Mucus in stool?	_____	_____
26. Rectal itching?	_____	_____
27. Vaginal itching?	_____	_____
28. Burning of penis?	_____	_____
29. Drainage of female urinary system?	_____	_____
30. Urinary urgency or frequency?	_____	_____
31. Burning upon urination?	_____	_____
32. Dark circles under eyes (shiners)?	_____	_____
33. Diminished sexual performance?	_____	_____

CHAPTER 15

Epstein-Barr Virus
and Chronic Fatigue
and Immune Dysfunction Syndrome

A NATIONAL PROBLEM

IN THE PAST TEN years, the medical community has focused growing attention on an illness that has come to be known as Chronic Fatigue and Immune Dysfunction Syndrome (CFIDS). Although the true number of its victims is unknown, thousands and thousands of people are reported to be suffering from a complex assortment of symptoms associated with this illness.

CFIDS usually affects persons in their early thirties. However, there are sufferers from those in their teens to a few in their seventies who are severely incapacitated. The syndrome occurs three times more often in females than in males.

❧ PREVIOUS DIAGNOSIS

Initially labeled Epstein-Barr Virus, the disease is generally traced to an epidemic of long-term fatigue accompanied by flulike symptoms. The first official reporting was in 1985, near Lake Tahoe, Nevada.

Until a few years ago, members if the medical community theorized that a common disease known as infectious mononucleosis, caused by the Epstein-Barr Virus, had been converted from its normally short-term, acute stage to a chronic, long-term sickness, encompassing a different set of symptoms. It sometimes lasted for years, with some people never recovering. Researchers subsequently found that approximately 90 percent of American adults have antibodies to mononucleosis whether or not they ever displayed symptoms of the disease.

❧ HHV-6 Virus

Today it is believed that Epstein-Barr Virus may be only one of many causes of CFIDS. A virus called HHV-6 may be another of the responsible agents. The disease is apparently based on reactivation of an old latent infection, by a stressful circumstance, by another virus, or even another illness.

❧ Overwhelming Exhaustion

Earlier the disease complex was appropriately titled "Chronic Fatigue Syndrome," since fatigue is the predominant complaint of its victims. This is not just ordinary tiredness, but exhaustion so overwhelming and of such long duration that lack of energy completely dominates and controls the victim's entire lifestyle. Interestingly, one physician's study recognized that 45 percent of all patients seeking medical attention today in the United States complain about some degree of fatigue. Obviously this represents a large national problem.

Along with fatigue, almost all CFIDS patients complain of generalized muscle aches, recurrent sore throats, and swollen lymph nodes. Another persistent problem that causes considerable concern is mental confusion and memory loss. They complain that their thinking is unclear, that they suddenly are unable to concentrate or perform tasks they could previously complete with ease. Balancing a checkbook, making phone calls, or remembering names and numbers requires a major effort. At times their fear over mental confusion and the resulting loss of self-confidence leads to neurosis.

Frequently CFIDS patients experience chest pain and palpitations and, at times, become convinced they have a serious cardiac condition. Quite often there are severe sleep disturbances, either insomnia or excessive sleep patterns. In the latter the patient may sleep as many as 18 hours a day and still feel tired.

웱 MEDICAL SYSTEM DENIES THE PROBLEM

Although it appears there are a large number of people experiencing this group of similar symptoms—and the quantity is growing rapidly—standard medical testing has failed to pinpoint a specific cause for their ills. Therefore the traditional medical system has largely denied or ignored the entire problem. A large segment of this expanding population of sick people has been told that the disease represents a syndrome that simply does not exist and that it is all in their minds, a psychological, not an organic, problem.

To make matters worse, even with the few doctors who have taken time to listen and recognize that, indeed, there is a serious problem, their response to the suffering patient is that there is no specific treatment or cure. The best they usually offer are generalities and platitudes, such as telling patients to avoid stress and to get more rest.

Evidence of the sufferers' resultant frustration is the more than 250 support groups that have been formed nationwide. Participants help one another deal with this baffling illness and pressure medical science into acknowledging that their symptoms do, indeed, represent a real disease.

웱 DIAGNOSIS

Diagnosis is made in several ways. First, identify active resurgence of the HHV-6 Virus. However, performing this test is usually impractical because of the cost and difficulty of obtaining the test. A test measuring T & B cell subsets is quite helpful, particularly in monitoring the disease as the immunity mechanisms may be affected. An MRI scan of the brain may reveal lesions in the subcortical region. There is now a profile of symptoms to help detect the presence of CFIDS. A test to confirm this profile is found at the end of this chapter.

Some CFIDS patients may have periods when they are completely free of symptoms and seem to function normally until a stressor confronts them. Stressors involve extreme emotional circumstances, an associated disease or a viral infection, a physical accident in which body trauma occurs, or a significant affront to the immune system, such as in the case of exposure to a heavy dose of pesticides or chemicals. Other CFIDS patients are seemingly never free of their symptoms.

Many CFIDS victims are unable to continue working. The trauma of long-term illness, the frustration of extreme fatigue, and the lack of understanding by others combines to cause many to suffer added emotional and psychological problems.

Some patients' lives have been so completely disrupted that they have divorced, lost all their friends, and become totally reclusive. Such behavior is due, in part, to the inability to interact socially, another consequence of having little energy and possessing a feeling of hopelessness.

✄ ACCOMPANYING CONDITIONS

A most noteworthy finding of the syndrome is the existence of accompanying disease states. In my practice I have noted this trend, and though little has been mentioned in medical literature, I have carefully documented my findings of six accompanying conditions:

1. Thyroid dysfunction: A thyroid that is usually underactive. This is represented by symptoms of cold hands and feet, hair loss, poor fingernail growth, sluggish bowels, and fatigue.
2. Temporal mandibular joint problems: Usually diagnosed by pain in the region where the jawbone attaches and hinges to the skull. Some patients awaken in the morning feeling this pain, while others have discomfort when chewing.
3. Infection with parasites and fungus: In which many patients have recurrent infections caused by a yeast known medically as Candida albicans. It causes vaginal, skin, and bowel infections and is commonly found in persons who have impaired immune systems. Also, most surprisingly, one study in India found 65 percent of the people who suffered from Chronic Fatigue Syn-

drome were additionally diagnosed as having a bowel parasite infestation called Giardiasis. This parasite normally causes gastric upset, gas, and bloating, and digestive problems. It also saps the strength of the host and removes important nutrients, adding to the overall condition of fatigue. Parasite tests are not normally performed in doctors' offices in the United States and consequently a parasite infestation is often missed. In addition, finding a laboratory that is proficient at identifying parasites is difficult. (See Chapter 13, "Are We Parasitized?", and Chapter 14, "Yeast Infection and Its Effects on Our Health.")

4. Mitral Valve Prolapse: The incomplete closure of a heart valve, while not common to all CFIDS sufferers, is seen in roughly 25 to 30 percent of the cases, a little higher than the national average. This leads to symptoms of chest pain and palpitations.

5. Sugar Intolerance and Reactive Hypoglycemia: A condition in which the patient, at times, has very low blood sugar levels leading to confusion, fatigue, agitation, anxiety, and a craving for sugar.

6. Allergies and hypersensitivity: To many environmental pollens and reactions to foods that are ingested daily.

It should be noted that not every CFIDS patient has all six of these conditions; however most have three or four.

❧ IMMUNE SYSTEM DAMAGE

The most challenging aspect of CFIDS is the problem that results from our immune systems having been attacked, damaged, and disabled by exposure to environmental pollutants. In modern society we are subjected to many chemicals, such as pesticides and food additives; heavy metals such as lead, cadmium, copper, mercury, and aluminum; petroleum distillates and plastics with hydrocarbons; and drugs including antibiotics and pain killers. All of these substances disturb our natural body metabolism and interfere with normal, healthy chemical reactions.

As a result the immune system, acting as our defense system, is incapacitated to the degree that our body is unable to defend itself from common infections and chemicals. In many cases it reacts to these substances so severely as to cause disability. This is a growing problem. One study shows that 6.5 million people in the U.S. are suffering from secondary immune dysfunction.

🜚 TREATMENT

Allopathically, a variety of treatments have been tried. One popular treatment, the antiviral drug Acyclovir, does not appear to work and may actually cause serious neurological problems. Several antidepressant drugs have been used with only minor success.

So how is this condition reversed holistically? The first and most obvious step is to help heal the immune system by avoiding exposure to destructive pollutants.

The second step is to detoxify the body completely to remove pesticides, heavy metals, and parasites, including *Candida*. (See Appendix A, Cleansing)

The third step involves intravenous administration of vitamin C to destroy viruses and neutralize undesirable substances that cannot be removed with oral homeopathic remedies. There is much data that confirms that vitamin C, particularly in high doses, acts as an antiviral substance. Man and the guinea pig are the only mammals that have lost the ability to manufacture vitamin C internally. Consequently it must be consumed daily.

The fourth step is to rebuild the immune system and balance the endocrine system and hormones with proper nutrition and exercise. (See Chapter 8.)

A product called Adenosine phosphate, when injected, appears to naturally stimulate physical strength and accelerate the metabolism. By accelerating the Krebs Cycle, this product has been shown to produce increased energy and a sense of well-being.

Dietary programs that emphasize natural foods and high doses of pure amino acids are very beneficial. I specifically recommend Glutathione, a tri-peptide that is valued in protection and rebuilding of the liver. It protects the body against toxins, and is also said to promote healthy longevity.

Another very important step involves emotional recovery. This is accomplished through hypnotherapy and emotional and spiritual support. Recently I integrated a process called "psychoneuroimmunology" into my practice. This means discovering ways a patient can be encouraged to activate the brain to stimulate the immune system to operate at a higher, more efficient level.

At least 85 percent of my CFIDS patients who have followed this program have achieved a healthy state of being.

☙ CHRONIC FATIGUE SYNDROME ASSESSMENT

I use this assessment in the diagnosis of CFIDS as well as to evaluate whether the therapy is effective.

A case of chronic fatigue syndrome must fulfill:

1. Both of the major criteria listed below; and
2. Either 2 or more of the 3 Physical Examination Criteria listed below and 6 or more of the Minor Symptom Criteria listed, or 8 or more of the Minor Symptom Criteria listed. Several of the Less Frequent Symptoms may also be present.
3. Symptom Criteria: The symptoms must have begun at or after the onset of increased fatigue and must have persisted or occurred over a period of at least six months.

MAJOR SYMPTOM CRITERIA	Before Therapy		After Therapy	
	YES	NO	YES	NO
1. A new onset of persistent or relapsing debilitating fatigue that does not resolve with bed rest.	___	___	___	___
2. Reduces daily activity by 50% for at least six months.	___	___	___	___

PHYSICAL EXAMINATION CRITERIA:	YES	NO	YES	NO
1. Low-grade fever (oral temperature 99.7-101.5°F)	___	___	___	___
2. Nonexudative pharyngitis (sore throat with no pus or discharge)	___	___	___	___
3. Palpable or tender cervical or axillary lymph nodes (<2 cm in diameter)	___	___	___	___

	Before Therapy		After Therapy	
MINOR SYMPTOM CRITERIA	YES	NO	YES	NO
1. Abrupt onset of complaints				
2. Muscle weakness				
3. Mild fever				
4. Sore throat				
5. Sleep disturbances				
6. Fatigue after exercise				
7. Generalized headaches				
8. Painful lymph nodes				
9. Neurophysiologic complaints				
10. Muscle pain				
11. Moving joint pain				
TOTALS				

LESS FREQUENT SYMPTOMS	YES	NO	YES	NO
1. Symptoms worsen with exhaustion				
2. Alcohol intolerance				
3. Unusual headaches				
4. Medication sensitivity				
5. Confusion in thinking				
6. Memory loss – memory sequential				
7. Spatial disorganization				
TOTALS				

CHAPTER 16

Holistic Approach to Memory Improvement

OUR BRAIN

OUR BRAIN orchestrates our behavior and bodily actions. It represents our survival, our creativity, our very existence. Memory is a function of the brain and helps us survive in a complex world.

Given normal environmental and heredity influences, the brain experiences growth or regeneration until approximately age 28. Afterwards degeneration slowly begins, accelerating as we age. An inadequate or poor circulatory system contributes to this degeneration by providing the brain with diminished supplies of oxygen, vitamins, minerals, and other essentials.

A study by Cutler and Grams published in the Journal of Gerontology describes factors that affect memory loss. The major factors evaluated and found significant were: age, gender, educational attainment, visual and auditory functional states, perceived changes in health, and the number of functional limitations. This study provided a comprehensive approach to understanding memory.

Obviously, the older we get the more possibilities exist that our memory can become diminished. As we age, our bodies degenerate and experience literally years of accumulation of toxins — heavy metals, pesticides, and other chemicals so prevalent in our society. Lack of nutrition and accumulated toxins may be directly responsible for brain degeneration and memory loss.

Aging, however, does not necessarily have to result in memory loss. According to Cutler's study, many aged persons have no significant memory loss. It was found that undertaking certain life-style changes may improve memory. For instance, memory can be enhanced by preventing damage to brain cells and therefore eliminating premature aging and senility.

It appears females are slightly more affected by memory loss than males, which may only be a reflection of the greater longevity of women. Also, more educated individuals may take better care of their health and have access to improved nutrition, so more educated people suffer less memory loss as time goes on.

Also, perceived changes in health showed a dramatic relationship with memory. Those who felt their health had improved during the previous year had significant improvement in memory. Conversely, persons who perceived that their health deteriorated reflected a decline in memory. Therefore, our belief system, coupled with feelings of well being, can enhance memory capacity. Wellness training, including exercise and behavior modification, may have a secondary benefit of improving memory.

According to the study, the last significant factor influencing memory is the number of functional limitations. Activities examined in this study included walking a quarter mile, carrying heavy packages, and kneeling. Closely akin to these measurements are states of visual and auditory acuity. Not surprising, the study found that the more normal physical functions one possesses, the better the memory. The converse was also true.

A correlation was also shown between poor hearing and poor memory, though poor hearing does not always reflect poor memory. While there seemed to be a relationship between poor vision and poor memory, it was not so apparent as with hearing.

Regular exercise and a healthy life-style contribute to good circulation and cellular nutrition that lead to a feeling of well being and, ultimately, results in better memory.

❦ HOLISTIC APPROACH

Fortunately when there is evidence of memory loss there are nutrients and medications that can make a difference. Here I list only those that have low side effects and are generally considered safe.

Choline

The brain requires acetylcholine for nerve impulses to travel from cell to cell transmitting messages to various sections of the brain and other vital body parts. If acetylcholine has been destroyed or insufficient amounts are produced, then it is necessary to replace the acetylcholine. Choline acts as a building block for the chemical acetylcholine. One of the best sources of choline is phosphatidyl choline. Vitamin B-5 (pantothenic acid) helps convert choline to acetylcholine.

Gerovital or GH-3

Discovered by Dr. Anna Aslan from Rumania, this substance has been known for years as an antiaging product. It is primarily made up of procaine, normally used as an anesthetic. Procaine rapidly breaks down into P.A.B.A., a vitamin, and DMAE, a memory enhancing drug that also increases acetylcholine levels in the brain.

Lucidril

The chemical name of this drug is centrophenoxine and has been widely used in Europe with success, according to Dr. Ross Pelton in his book Mind Food and Smart Pills. It reverses the aging process and removes abnormal fatty deposits, called lipofuscin, from around nerve cells. Lipofuscin, accumulating with age, represents a breakdown of metabolic substances and blocks normal nerve impulses. Lucidril has been shown to improve conditions such as mental confusion and loss of memory.

Piracetam

Widely used in Europe and Mexico, piracetam is said to enhance learning and memory. It also protects the brain against oxygen starvation, protects against memory loss from physical injury and chemical poisoning, and promotes movement of information between the left and right hemispheres of the brain. Remember, the right hemisphere controls artistic, intuitive, and creative abilities while the left hemisphere orchestrates the rational, reasoning aspect of our mind and directs our speech center if we are right handed. This drug creates better assimilation of knowledge.

Given simultaneously, the effects of piracetam and choline are greatly increased, dramatically improving memory and data retention. This relationship is called synergism, which means that together their positive effects are increased.

Hydergine
This has been used in the United States for several years to increase blood supply to the brain by removing lipofuscin and promoting free radical scavenging. Hydergine, therefore, improves memory, reasoning, and intelligence. I have prescribed it for a number of years and find it is safe and results in improved mental functioning after about four months of use. Because a close colleague, Dr. Ronald Lesko, D.O., Ph.D., published some original research on Hydergine, I am aware of a secondary, previously unreported effect of the drug—it reverses impotency in some males.

Eldepryl
This exceptional product stimulates a portion of the brain known as the substantive nigra. It causes the production of the chemical dopamine, which maintains healthy brain cells. If brain cells are weak or old and ready to die, eldepryl can bring them back to life. It can produce alertness, mobility, memory improvement, and a sense of well being. It is effective in treating Alzheimer's, Parkinson's, depression, fatigue, blepharspasm, peripheral neuropathy, tremors, and senility. It is said to also promote longevity.

Vitamins, Minerals, and Herbs
Vitamins have long been known to enhance memory and provide cellular protection. Free radicals, the final metabolites of fat, damage brain cells and are thought to be the major cause of atherosclerosis (hardening of the arteries) and premature aging. Certain vitamins protect

cells from free radicals and prolong the functions and life of the brain. The most common are vitamins A, C, E, and the mineral selenium (remember ACES). These are traditionally called free radical scavengers because of their ability to pick up and deactivate oxygen free radicals. One should take these anti-oxidants, as they are also called, daily due to the large amounts of harmful substances we ingest and breath.

Many herbs stimulate mental activity, too. Ginseng, in particular, improves memory, learning, and concentration. Ginkgo biloba is another brain stimulator.

Chelation

All of the above therapies are considered noninvasive. I feel, however, that when the patient's condition has deteriorated significantly, a more aggressive treatment should be used to improve memory.

Poor memory may be the result of years of improper diet and poor environment including exposure to heavy metals such as lead, mercury, and aluminum. These metals can accumulate in brain cells and interfere with our thinking process. Aluminum, for instance, has recently been identified in the brain cells of many Alzheimer's victims and is believed to be related to the high incidence of the disease in the elderly.

Chelation therapy rapidly brings the patient to a state of good health by increasing oxygen flow and improving circulation in the brain and all other areas of the body. Chelation therapy is a fast, effective way to remove unwanted plaque and open blood vessels. (See Chapter 9.)

Hypnotherapy

Lastly, as the Cutler study states, perceived belief of health plays a major role in memory. Consequently, a therapy that promotes a healthy attitude will have a dramatic effect. I have noted good results from hypnotherapy, performed in my office and followed by the patient listening to the taped session at home as needed. Many patients report they feel better, have a more positive outlook on life, and notice improved memory because of the hypnosis.

Overall, greater positive results are achieved by a combination of the above therapies, properly designed and monitored by a physician.

REFERENCES:

Cutler, Stephen J. and Armin E. Grams. "Correlates of Self-Reported Everyday Memory Problems," From *Journal of Gerontology: Social Sciences*, 1988, Vol. 43, No. 3, p. 582-90.

Pelton, Ross, M.D. *Mind Food and Smart Pills*. San Diego: T & R, 1986.

CHAPTER 17

Reversing Arthritis, Inflammation, and Disease of the Joints and Spine

WHAT KIND OF A JOINT IS THIS?

THERE ARE VARIOUS types of joint diseases—inflammatory, non-inflammatory, and others. Inflammatory types include rheumatoid arthritis, gouty arthritis, Rieter's syndrome, systemic lupus erythematosus (SLE), scleroderma, ankylosing spondylitis (AS), and colitis/enteritis-related arthritis.

The noninflammatory arthritis types include osteoarthritis, traumatic arthritis, and osteochondromatosis.

Other pathologies we see are a bacterial invasion of the joints and tumors or blood entering the joint and creating an unusual type of joint damage. However, the latter is rare and will not be discussed in this book.

The pathology seen at the joint level includes inflammation, fluid formation, and ultimately calcification, which may involve surrounding tissue, including cartilage, bone, ligaments, and tendons. In chronic conditions the entire joint may be calcified or fibrosed and fixed or, as it is called in the medical books, ankylosed. Nodules are also sometimes formed under the skin. These are also found in the muscle and surrounding sac and valves of the heart, lungs, around the brain and spinal cord, and in the spleen and larynx of the throat. In fact, during autopsy, inflammation of the heart is seen in 25 to 40 percent of the patients that have some form of arthritis.

Other lesions found in arthritis include small vessel inflammation, pulmonary fibrosis, and disturbances of the skeletal muscle as well as the lymph nodes. Consequently, it is clear that this disease represents a serious systemic problem affecting many parts of the body.

Diagnosis

Diagnosis is made by a thorough history and examination. However, x-rays may be very valuable in confirming the diagnosis and the degree of joint involvement. Occasionally CT-scans and MRIs may be utilized.

Laboratory findings are very valuable in diagnosing and monitoring the progress of the disease. Measuring such parameters as sedimentation rate, IgM antibodies, latex fixation test, ANA titers, presence of uric acid crystals, and HLA-B27 antigens is important.

Treatment

The treatments for these diseases varies, of course, depending upon the type of disease and stage of development. First, I will discuss general principles of physical management.

Bed rest

In all cases of significant spinal problems, a trial of bed rest is suggested as a first line of treatment. Usually a minimum of two weeks is recommended.

Physical Therapy

There are several types of physical therapy used for arthritis, including: "passive range of motion," wherein someone other than the patient moves the joints; "active range of motion," in which the patient does the moving; and "isometric," in which the muscle is contracted but the joint is hardly moved at all. All of these therapies help to strengthen the body.

For low back problems—a very common condition—it is critical to exercise responsibly. One important procedure is to strengthen the abdominal muscles, thereby taking some weight off and resting the back muscles and consequently sharing the load. This can be done by performing sit-ups.

Hydrotherapy

Exercise performed in the water, thereby supporting the weight of the individual—is very effective. Also, the agitation of the water creates a gentle massaging action. When mineral salts are added an additional benefit is obtained as these are absorbed through the skin and both strengthen and relax the muscles.

Next, heat or cold packs can be applied. In some cases, heat is better; in others, cold works better. For example, when treating acute inflammation due to trauma, cold compresses usually act to keep the swelling down and relieve the pain during the first 24 hours. After the first 24 hours, heat packs usually work better by improving circulation to the area. Heat packs are also more effective on chronic inflammation.

Massage

Massage improves the circulation and removes congestion of the tissue. It also improves the lymphatic circulation and removes toxins. Another benefit is that it encourages the release of muscles that are in spasm, therefore getting them back into proper motion. Also, I have observed that when pressure is applied properly it can lead to the break up of small crystals of calcium and other minerals. This causes the pain to subside and helps the circulatory system remove these deposits.

Medicines

Specific medicinal intervention includes the popular nonsteroidal, anti-inflammatory drugs, commonly called NSAIDS. A few of the more common drugs are Indocin, Motrin, Naprosyn, Feldene, Meclomen, Vicodin, and Clinoril. They are taken by billions of people in this country and are heavily promoted by the physicians and the pharmaceutical companies. Obviously huge profits are made on these drugs! Each year several new "arthritis" drugs are marketed by the pharmaceutical industry. Unfortunately, these drugs do not cure, but only temporarily relieve the pain and reduce swelling.

The problem with these drugs, other than their high cost, is that they can be dangerous to us, particularly when taken over long periods of time. First, these drugs can cause bleeding of the stomach and bowels that could be life threatening. Worse, from the perspective of the arthritis sufferer, one of the drugs, Indocin, appears to actually accelerate the action of joint destruction. This is according to a study done in Oslo, Norway, and reported by Dr. Julian Whitaker in his June 1993 newsletter, "Dr. Julian Whitaker's Health & Healing." So ironically, here are medications that are expensive, dangerous, and actually cause us more problems if taken for long periods of time.

Another commonly used drug is called a steroid or cortisone and is equally detrimental. If taken for a only a short time, such as weeks, it may not be too hazardous and may actually be beneficial. However, if taken over a long period of time, it can cause serious side effects. These effects again include gastrointestinal bleeding in addition to hormonal upsets. An example may be the production of diabetes and the suppression of the adrenal glands that protect the body from stress. The adrenals may be so severely damaged over long-term therapy that they quit functioning completely, causing depression and even shock if the cortisone treatment is ceased suddenly. Also, these drugs help promote the removal of calcium from the bone causing premature osteoporosis (brittle bones), in which the fracture of a bone could occur even with minimal movement or trauma—a very serious situation.

So What Is the Answer?

The answer is to approach arthritis and joint problems from a more direct intervention. Understanding the root cause of the problem helps to focus our therapies. There are general but very important things that we may do:

Diet

There is much evidence that diet and our assimilation of food may be a major factor in the cause of joint disease. One very good example is that a number of serious diseases of the bowel, including ulcerative colitis, regional enteritis, and Whipples' disease, have accompanying diseases that are undistinguishable from rheumatoid arthritis. Furthermore, when the bowel disease is cured, the arthritis condition improves as well.

How does this work? I have already described how the health of the digestive tract and specifically the bowel integrity affects what we absorb into our systems. If the natural filtering system of the bowel lining is disrupted then many large substances are able to enter our bodies. Therefore, if instead of having three-angstrom size openings in our bowel, we have 30- or 300-angstrom size openings, long chain polypeptides could be admitted into our systems. As mentioned earlier, polypeptides activate a chain of events that challenge the immune system and the liver detoxifying mechanisms. The proteins and other products that survive our defense mechanisms often end up in the joint spaces. Here, an inflammatory reaction occurs, and if left untreated could ultimately cause pain and destruction of the joint. The final result is fibrosis and calcification of the joints and surrounding tissues.

Consequently healing the intestinal tract with vitamins, minerals, and homeopathic remedies is a starting place. This is followed by the reestablishment of the normal bowel flora with acidophilus.

Next, avoid those foods that you are sensitive to. Identify these food through a food allergy blood exam. Usually after eight weeks of avoidance, sensitive foods can be introduced back into the diet, one at a time. Be certain to keep a strict food diary to identify all symptoms produced by these foods (See "Food Response Assessment" at the end of Chapter 10.)

EDTA / Chelation

Another treatment is chelation. As mentioned, the process of chelation removes excess pathological calcium from joints and surrounding tissues. EDTA (the primary protein used in chelation) also removes heavy metals and many toxins and other chemicals. (See

Chapter 9 for more on chelation.) If the problem is spurs or other calcification in the spine, then chelation, along with gentle manipulation, may help.

Glucosamine

Glucosamine, when given at the level of three to six capsules daily is a remarkable treatment for arthritis. It reduces joint pain, rebuilds joints and connective tissue, and reduces joint inflammation. As already mentioned, a study cited by Dr. Julian Whitaker in his newsletter, showed that it works in both rheumatoid arthritis and osteoarthritis. Most important, it is safe.

I have found that the essential oil birch is beneficial in the treatment of joint pain. By rubbing a few drops topically over the joint, pain and swelling were dramatically reduced in many cases.

Electro-Auricular Acupuncture

One way to reduce pain simply and naturally is electro-auricular acupuncture. This procedure uses low-voltage electricity on acupuncture points in the ear that correspond to the points in the body that are diseased with arthritis. I have observed severe pain disappear in a matter of minutes and stay away for weeks and occasionally indefinitely after a single treatment. In some cases, several treatments are required. Of course, there is essentially no risk with this therapy.

Colchicine

While not specifically in the category of arthritis, herniated or ruptured discs in the lower back are a serious problem often associated with arthritis. In the case of herniated spinal disks, colchicine has provided remarkable benefits. Colchicine is one of the most powerful anti-inflammatory medications known. According to research performed by Dr. Michael R. Rash and published in *The Journal of Neurological and Orthopaedic Medicine and Surgery*, colchicine, injected intravenously, rapidly reverses disc disease even when other therapies have failed. While surgery is used in many cases, because of the expense and prolonged recovery time, I feel that colchicine should be tried first. Be aware that in some cases scar tissue formed post-surgically, not a disc, recreates the original pain, making surgery necessary again, but it is much more difficult to achieve success the second time.

In some cases I have seen dramatic results with one or two shots of colchicine, which causes the nerve irritation to rapidly subside and the protruding ruptured disc to shrink. I have literally seen patients who had experienced years of crippling pain get up and walk, without pain, after several injections.

Also, good results are being obtained in the case of lower spinal disc problems with a procedure called "facet nerve block." The process, developed by Dr. Norman Shealy of the Shealy Institute, involves an injection of colchicine into the area of the spinal nerves. This, in some cases, removes the back pain indefinitely. It is a very safe procedure.

Naturally, every therapy should be individualized according to the patient and condition. This is especially true of such a diverse disease as arthritis and associated joint and spinal problems.

REFERENCES:

Rash, Michael R., M.D. "Colchicine Use in 6000 Patients with Disk Disease & Other Related Resistantly Painful Spinal Disorders." From *The Journal of Neurological and Orthopaedic Medicine and Surgery*, December 1989, Vol. 10, Issue 4.

Whitaker, Julian, M.D. "Dr. Julian Whitaker's Health & Healing." Newsletter: June 1993, Vol. 3, No. 6. Potomac, MD: Phillips Publishing, Inc.

CHAPTER 18

Healing AIDS

A POLITICAL, SOCIOECONOMIC, MEDICAL DISEASE

FOURTEEN MILLION PEOPLE have been infected by AIDS (Acquired Immune Deficiency Syndrome). AIDS is a political and socioeconomic disease as well as a medical problem. AIDS is a disease of the body, mind, spirit, and emotions. AIDS is a psychological disease and a physical one. Some symptoms are mental suffering, denial, guilt, anger, confusion, depression, and memory loss. In part, this is due to a biochemical imbalance that affects the nervous system. AIDS is a multifaceted, complex disease.

The intestine secretes a substance called VIP (Vasoactive Intestinal Polypeptide). It is released during REM (rapid eye movement) sleep and causes people to dream more. It is also secreted during the day and serves as a growth factor for neurons, producing dendrites and axons, helping the neurons to grow. This counteracts the action of the AIDS virus that causes stripping of dendrites and the ultimate death of these nerves.

In the case of AIDS, there is a basic immune problem as well. When a virus attacks the immune system and cripples or destroys its function, any germ that the patient comes in contact with could overwhelm the immune system. In many cases this is so profound that death ensues. However, it is usually not immediate, but takes years to totally destroy the immune system.

AIDS is usually transmitted by sexual contact. There seems to be two other factors that could contribute to the disease:

1. Excessive stress;
2. Simultaneous excessive use of chemical substances, primarily but not necessarily, illicit drugs.

There are exceptions to these rules. Namely, the disease can be transmitted through the placenta to newborn children, by way of blood transfusions, infected needles, or intravenous drug users, or by contact with contaminated blood.

According to Dr. Laurence Badgley, "As with any immune problem, treatment is most successful if both preventive measures and immune-strengthening procedures are taken simultaneously." The same ideas for strengthening the immune system as defined in Chapter 10, "Allergies and the Immune System," apply to AIDS.

ALTERNATIVE THERAPIES

An underground movement has been formed by individuals with the disease who are taking personal responsibility. These AIDS patients have sought, investigated, and used alternative therapies themselves, doing this usually without their physicians' involvement. This is because many patients have seen AIDS sufferers treated with mainstream drugs and therapies, usually costing hundreds of thousands of dollars, only to ultimately end in terrible personal suffering and death.

The problem is two fold. First, many people have a mind set that any drug or therapy outside of the establishment (pharmaceutical companies, hospitals, and universities) has no validity or benefit. Second, the process of getting approval for many natural products and therapies is cost prohibitive. The expenditure usually runs as high as $200 million per product for FDA approval. Obviously an herb that sells for ten cents per capsule with a profit of two cents has no potential for recouping that original expense, so there is no profit motive to have it tested and approved. This is not true in other countries where the high cost of government approval does not exist.

Many AIDS patients are discovering that what U.S. pharmaceutical companies have to offer falls short. They are consequently led to investigate alternative therapies.

Some patients have seen a positive turn around in their health after using these alternative therapies. They have obviously informed other AIDS victims and eventually an underground source of knowledge and therapies has sprung up. Many drugs that have proven efficacious and safe in other countries are finding their way to these AIDS sufferers and with good results.

Keep in mind that many people have suffered and even more have died because of the resistance of many professionals to be open and look at simple alternatives. Many therapies do not fit the current medical models but are nevertheless beneficial.

Peptide T

One such therapy, which has been discovered and is still being tested, is an amino-acid peptide called Peptide T. When administered to an AIDS patient it immediately blocks the advance of the disease.

It was discovered by Candice Pert, Ph.D., in 1985 at the National Institute of Mental Health. It was tested on eight cases of terminal AIDS patients in Sweden and on four advanced cases in Los Angeles several years ago. Improvement occurred in most of these patients even though their conditions were advanced.

The pharmaceutical company Burroughs Wellcome initially agreed to produce this product in the United States. However, according to Pert, after imposing a two-year gag rule while researching the efficacy of using this new peptide, Burroughs Wellcome decided to produce a different anti-AIDS drug.

Interestingly enough, this new peptide product binds the receptor sites of cells, preventing the AIDS virus from attaching to them. Consequently, this is a nontoxic treatment.

Extracorporeal photopheresis

Another treatment that deserves further evaluation is extracorporeal photopheresis. A study published in Annuals of Internal Medicine 1990 revealed that five AIDS patients treated with ultraviolet light showed a positive result. While this study represented a small group, the results were still hopeful. After 14 months two of them were found negative for HIV. The other two revealed a significant improvement in quality of life. The remaining patient dropped out of the study on his own.

Center for 21st Century Medicine

While head of a clinic in Los Angeles, the Center for 21st Century Medicine, Dr. Joan Priestly, had success treating AIDS. Dr. Priestly presented her results to the international AIDS conference in China, Italy, and Germany. This is a balanced program, and she has seen prolonged survival and reversal of the disease.

Dr. Priestly's program is as follows:
1. High doses of vitamins and minerals, particularly beta-carotene, C, and E, taken both intravenously and orally;
2. Garlic, large doses taken orally;
3. Acetylcysteine in high doses;
4. Acidophilus, taken orally;
5. Quercetin, a form of bioflavonoid, taken orally;
6. St. John's wart herb, taken orally;
7. Aloe vera (brand name R-Pure Aloe or Aloe Magic), taken orally;
8. Dinitrochloro benzene lotion, applied weekly to the skin;
9. Co Enzyme Q 10, taken orally;
10. DHEA (dehydroepiandrosterone), taken orally;
11. Zinc (maximum dose 100 mg daily), taken orally;
12. L-Carnitine, taken orally;
13. Opti-weight maintenance supplement.

Obviously it is a program that works as she has treated many patients with success. Please note that Dr. Priestly recently moved her practice to Alaska.

Our system is in desperate need of change. We as a nation must develop more compassion and begin to practice the art as well as the science of medicine.

REFERENCES:

Badgley, Laurence, MD. *Healing AIDS Naturally.* San Bruno, CA: Human Energy Press, 1987.

Moyers, Bill. *Healing and the Mind.* New York: Doubleday, 1993.

CHAPTER 19

The Non-Disease Illness

FEELING BAD

A PATIENT ONCE CAMe to me with numerous complaints. Her major problem was fatigue. She also complained of lack of strength, muscle aches, a vague feeling of anxiety and fear. She also felt that she was being affected by fumes of all kinds, including smoke and most perfumes. And she said that she could not tolerate any medications as their effects always seemed quite strong and persisted for days. Even the smallest dose seemed to cause terrible side effects.

This patient had been having these problems for over a year and the symptoms had just been getting worse. During that time she had consulted four physicians and none had given her any encouragement. In fact, only two of the physicians had even bothered ordering a routine blood chemistry test, and they ultimately announced that there was nothing wrong with her. When she insisted that she did have a problem, they suggested that she see a psychiatrist.

Two years earlier, after the persistence of a chronic bronchial infection, this patient had been on antibiotic therapy for several months. She had also been on anti-ulcer medication for a suspected ulcer, and she had never quite felt the same since.

Some medications inactivate the cytochrome P450 mechanism of the liver. The function of this enzyme is to inactivate many drugs including caffeine. I agreed that her life was not in immediate danger from this disease. However, she was most assuredly made miserable by her symptoms. She had to adapt to a lifestyle where she tried desperately to avoid those things that she had already identified as not good for her.

❧ SELF-IMPOSED PRISON

Her self-imposed life-style was so limiting that at times she felt that she was imprisoned. Yet none of the physicians who had previously seen her performed a test to measure her first line of protective defense—the ability of her bowel tract to filter the toxic products she had ingested. Nor did they measure the liver detoxification function—the ability of her liver to successfully neutralize toxins. This is the second line of defense to protect her body from numerous toxins, medications, and stimulants such as caffeine and other foods. Had they done these tests they would have found that her system was on the verge of eminent breakdown leading to some more serious disease. Her defense mechanisms were seriously compromised by medications and toxins. Her final symptoms were triggered by stress that kept her body in a continuous alarm state, further depleting her detoxifying and immune defending systems.

Recommending that she see a psychiatrist made matters worse. Her husband and other family members had grown tired of hearing her complain and when a nonphysical problem was officially proclaimed they felt she was malingering to avoid her responsibilities. "You look well," they used to say. The last physician's recommendation solidified their opinions and everyone pretty much sealed her fate, giving her very little desire to search for further help. However, deep inside she was convinced this was not originally a mental or psychological condition, but the result of a physical illness.

A Real Illness

Consequently she sought me out after hearing from a friend that I dealt with similar difficult metabolic problems. After I took a history and gave her a physical exam and laboratory studies, including a bowel permeability test and a thorough liver function test, it became clear to me that she was suffering from "leaky gut syndrome." This is a disease in which the bowel abnormally admits large particles of chemicals, toxins, and foods.

In addition, her liver function was so compromised that it could no longer neutralize these products and they began to attack her body systems. We quickly started therapy to detoxify her system and initiated products to rebuild her bowel lining, liver, and immune system.

Today this patient is doing fine. Her energy has returned to a high level and she is happy and healthy and now enjoys good family relationships.

Unfortunately, there are many more patients who have similar problems and go through emotional and mental trauma just as this patient did. They are told by physicians that there is nothing wrong with them. Their conditions begin subtly. There are very few signs and blood tests to confirm the diagnosis early in the course of the disease. Usually doctors must depend heavily on the patient's history. In this busy world of medicine, there is much pressure to see many patients in a day and it is difficult to spend a lot of time with each patient. Nevertheless, in many cases, we must take the time to listen intently to the patient. Usually they will give us their own diagnosis.

Section Three
WHERE DO WE GO FROM HERE?

INTRODUCTION

IN THIS SECTION I summarize the process of health care and discuss what we can expect in the future and what we can do, both as individuals and as a nation, to shape medicine in the United States.

The government has its own ideas as to what needs to be done. I propose that this governmental concept is not necessarily what we as citizens really want nor what is best for us.

I go on to summarize the holistic movement and describe how it impacts us and fulfills our needs.

Chapter 20

Medicine: A Freedom of Choice?

A Time of Transition

E UROPE AND THE EASTERN BLOC countries have gone through many changes in recent years and are still in a state of flux. The desire for freedom and democracy is sweeping much of the world. However, the Middle East is still very unsettled. Tempers flare easily and the clarion call for moderation and restraint comes from many people who desire peace.

The world economy is in transition as well, with vast fortunes being made and lost overnight. For security and refuge, countries are joining together in economic unity as trade barriers are disbanded.

Perhaps the greatest change today is the explosion of communications by way of computers and the Internet. Many people all over the world can now easily and cheaply talk to each other. There are estimated to be from 50 to 60 million people on the Internet worldwide. The United States alone has approximately 35 million on the Internet, and information on virtually all topics can be obtained there. We are truly riding on the Information Superhighway.

Multi-level marketing (MLM) is one of the fastest growing industries in the world. One of the reasons for this is that success depends on networking and communication to others about multi-level products.

Much money is being made in MLM, which is also creating financial independence for many persons as well as many new millionaires. Communication through MLM has reached an incredible level. People are talking to each other about taking personal responsibility for their health. In a way, it is breaking the pattern of complete dependency on the medical profession. At least it is getting people to communicate with each other and at the most empowering them.

⚘ THE HEALTH CRISIS

The field of medicine and health is no exception for these international "winds of change." The cost of medicine is running close to $1 trillion annually in the United States. At the rate of over $1 million per minute, this is second to nothing, not even food prices, in its rapid increase, according to the former chief of the U.S. Health and Human Resources Department, Joseph Califono.

With the impact of AIDS in the last two decades, the entire medical system has been significantly affected, requiring a new examination of our health-care approach.

We have a major challenge in medicine today. It is the appearance of killer microbes all around us. One recent magazine's cover story asks "Are we losing the war against infectious disease?" It seems this assault comes from two places. First, there is an appearance of new microbes, viruses, fungi, bacteria, and prozoan forms that are seriously affecting the health of people around the world. Second, old microbes are resurfacing.

Some of the new we are seeing microbes can reproduce in just 20 minutes. They can be very pathogenic. Some are fatal within hours after a person becomes infected. There are new microbes called flesh-eating bacteria that literally consume the flesh in hours.

New parasites are presently attacking peoples' gastrointestinal tracts, causing dysentery. An example of this is the protozoa Cyclospora, which produces diarrhea, vomiting, weight loss, fatigue, and muscle aches when it is consumed. It was believed that this parasite was brought in on the surface of fresh strawberries that were imported from South America.

An interesting fact about cyclospora is that it was rare to find its existence anywhere when I was reviewing the world literature in 1992. Where did it and other new bugs come from? Scientists propose two important theories. First, because of rapid reproduction of these microbes and also because of many toxins in our environment this produces rapid genetic changes of the life forms. The second concept is that the microbes have resided quietly for generations in our rain forests. Once the rain forests are disturbed these microbes are free to travel throughout the planet.

The recent cover story of USA Today was entitled, "Ancient Ills Return with a Vengeance." According to the story many illnesses that we thought were gone are recycling again to become serious health threats.

As mentioned earlier in this book, we are seeing a resurgence of many old diseases. This is due to three factors; frequent air travel, a lack of vigilance that is opening the door and allowing these microbes to come in, and antibiotic resistance. Because they do multiply so rapidly, they can change their character quickly and rebuild new genetic structure.

The past chief of the FDA, David A. Kessler, stated that the number one problem in health care today is the rapid emergence of new antibiotic-resistant microbes. So we must find new and natural projects to combat these 21st century invaders.

Another situation exists: The number of persons reaching the age of 65 years and older is significantly increasing. Because of their age, this group as a whole requires more medical support with hospitalization and expensive medical procedures.

ALTERNATIVE SOLUTIONS

I know that alternative therapies have many of the answers to these major health crises. Even though the word "alternative" is commonly used in the press, most modern physicians use the word "complementary," as I do. This term clearly implies the inclusion of standard allopathic medicine, but certainly does not consider it to be an exclusive approach to health care. It stresses the use of other natural therapies.

⚘ ALTERNATIVE BIASES

However, with the reality of major health problems confronting the American public, and with no easy solutions in the offing, I am amazed at the resistance and negativism expressed by the power structure of medicine and the popular press.

Many physicians are holistic in their approach to medicine, looking at the whole person in all dimensions, including the body, mind, emotions, and spirit. In doing so, they evaluate the environment and family interactions including co-dependency. They also include stress and possible physical danger from school and work place and even more subtle situations, many of which are ignored by the average physician. In turn, they use modalities such as visualization, positive-thinking techniques, homeopathy, aromatherapy, herbal, acupuncture, manipulation, massage, nutrition, and orthomolecular therapy. They also use many other generally accepted therapies, including medications and surgery.

Unfortunately, because some of these therapies have been discovered only recently and are not taught in medical school, they are attacked by some medical boards, insurance companies, and some areas of the media. For example, in five years of medical school I received only 20 hours of nutritional education, indicating a major neglect of this important topic.

Pioneering physicians are often punished because of this bias against complementary modalities. For example, a nationally respected author and pediatrician had his medical license revoked when he recommended chiropractic treatment along with nutritional counseling for a childhood illness. The fact that the child he was treating was cured was of no consequence; it was the doctor's technique that concerned the medical board.

✺ NUTRITION AND HEALTH

It is well known that nutrition plays a major role in an individual's health. Serious degenerative diseases have been reversed by nutritionally balanced programs such as macrobiotics and vegetarian diets.

In 1980 the United States Senate published a report entitled "Nutrition and Mental Health: A Hearing Before the Select Committee on Nutrition and Humans' Needs." It concluded that many diseases such as depression, fatigue, schizophrenia, low blood sugar, and heavy metal toxicity may be caused by improper diet in addition to the presence of large amounts of toxic substances in our environment. The over-processing of foods was named as one of the causative factors. The report said that improving the diet as well as adding vitamins and minerals might be curative and could lead to dramatic changes in an individual's health. Yet this study has been largely ignored by the medical profession.

Because over the years American soils have become over-used and depleted of nutrients, in some cases our food does not contain adequate vitamins, minerals, and other essential nutrition. Attempts to replenish the soil with commercial fertilizers appear inadequate, as many of the nutrients simply are not replaced. In addition the policy of over-processing and refining food means people are not receiving full nutritional value from the food supply today. Add to this the increased nutrient requirements because of our increasingly polluted environment and the overall situation becomes worse. This is why the frequently made statement "If you eat a well-balanced diet you don't need to take vitamins and minerals" is so wrong! Considering the status of nutrition today, it should be obvious that many of us should take vitamins and mineral supplements daily.

People, other than ourselves, are making decisions about our health and most of the time our best interests are not really the main issue. For example, many food additives and chemicals that have no nutrient value and, in fact, are often detrimental to our health are found in our diet. Aspartame (NutraSweet) is a good example. Statistics reveal that more than 100 million persons currently use Aspartame and yet there were cases reported by H.J. Roberts, M.D., director of the Palm Beach Institute of Medical Research, Inc., that indicated that severe reactions may occur from consumption of this product. These include diminished vision or blindness, severe headaches, convulsions, profound confusion and memory loss, dizziness, extreme depression, fatigue, hives, rashes, hyperactivity, ringing in the ears, loss of diabetic control, weight gain or loss, joint pain, and insomnia or loss of sleep.

Dr. Roberts has received over 10,000 complaints from consumers of Aspartame and although he has informed the authorities of these concerns, nothing has been done by the government. One might receive insight as to why this is so by looking at how Aspartame was introduced into our diet through soft drinks, cereals, instant coffees and teas, desserts, and even vitamins as well as many other products.

First, we must realize that the FDA did not test the product, but accepted data from the manufacturer. In April 1981, the acting FDA commissioner, Arthur Hull Hayes, newly appointed by the Reagan administration, overruled the recommendations of the FDA scientists that "a liquid form should not be used." In fact the initial license issued in 1981 was for the dry form only because it was felt that the liquid form had too many side effects.

In 1983, however, the FDA approved Aspartame for use in carbonated beverages. According to the Palm Beach Institute for Medical Research, Inc., Commissioner Hayes resigned his post two months later and went to work for a firm that represents Searle's NutraSweet advertising account.

In the summer of 1984 the National Soft Drink Association prepared a 31 page protest against the use of Aspartame in carbonated beverages. Consequently they were assured that most people would only consume one soft drink daily as it is the cumulative effect that appeared to be detrimental. Of course this has proven to be incorrect; as we know many people consume numerous Aspartame-sweetened drinks daily, plus they receive Aspartame from other food sources.

Worse is the cavalier attitude of our governmental regulators who felt that in general, herbs and vitamins have no significant effects on the body. Consequently they have not bothered to establish guidelines and quality control standards for their manufacture and distribution. Recently, however, they have swung completely in the other direction. The FDA is attempting to classify herbs and vitamins as drugs that will require a prescription for their purchase!

In contrast, when a popular and profitable medication or surgical procedure fails or causes serious side effects, we accept that as part of the risk of therapy.

In many instances when a patient has exhausted his possibilities of standard therapy he may seek help from a physician who practices complementary medicine. However, if that therapy fails, the physician is quite often reprimanded and risks censorship and the possible loss of his license to practice. He may also be singled out and quite often suffers public criticism.

In the past as well, many of our early scientists and forefathers who dared to be different suffered much humiliation and in some cases were jailed and even put to death. Doctor Lister, the physician who dared to suggest that hospital rooms and equipment must be cleaned and that physicians must wash their hands between patients was ostracized and expelled from the hospital—because of his forethought and pioneering conclusions.

At first the inventor of the electrocardiogram was told that his discovery was nonsense and not beneficial. It took 25 years to be fully accepted, although now we routinely accept the EKG in our medical work-ups.

Many physicians in authority are either prejudiced by their training or fear chastisement from their colleagues who claim that complementary medicine has no therapeutic value. This fact makes obtaining research grants and federal assistance almost nonexistent in the holistic field. Obviously, it is time for this attitude to be reversed!

The issue here, also, is the patient's freedom to receive correct information and make his own choice as to the kind of health care he desires. This is an act of self-responsibility and allows people to function as mature adults with control over their lives.

Much good medical research is being suppressed because editors of major medical journals won't allow holistic data to be published. In addition to this, the board that regulates which publications are to be placed in the Library of Congress typically excludes holistic material. This keeps valuable reference material from the medical community.

The Constitution of the United States guarantees us the freedom to practice the religion of our choice, to speak out, to vote, to bear arms, but not to practice the freedom of choice when it comes to the decision of our own health care and medical destiny; that freedom has been excluded.

Surprisingly, many European countries do include this freedom in their constitutions. Homeopathy is one of the major types of medicine practiced in England, for example.

The medical trend should include more holistic approaches in health, according to the prestigious "Trend Analysis Program and Health Care of the Future," published 13 years ago by the American Council of Life Insurance.

In conclusion, the patient must have the ultimate decision-making ability concerning his health as well as his pursuit of happiness.

REFERENCES

The American Council of Life Insurance. "Trend Analysis Program and Health Care of the Future." Report: Spring, 1980.

The United States Senate. "Nutrition and Mental Health: A Hearing Before The Select Committee on Nutrition and Humans' Needs." Washington, D.C.: 1980.

The United States Senate. "Nutrition and Mental Health." Hearing before the Select Committee on Nutrition and Human Needs of the United States Senate, 95th Congress, Washington D.C.: June 22, 1977.

CHAPTER 21

The Holistic Approach to
Better Health and Higher Consciousness

A SYSTEM OF HEALTH CARE

I stated the following earlier in this book, but I feel that it needs to be emphasized: Holistic medicine is a system of health care that fosters a cooperative relationship between the physician and the patient and other involved health professionals heading toward an attunement of body, mind, and spirit. It particularly encourages the patients to take personal responsibility for their life-style and the primary way of accomplishing this task is through education.

I see the goal of the new holistic movement as providing solutions to the afflictions of modern civilization. The primary modalities used by this approach are nutrition, homeopathy, aromatherapy, ortho-molecular medicine, structural integration, behavioral modification, exercise, improvement of our environment, and, particularly, spiritual attunement.

Experience now shows that the major etiological factor in modern diseases is a substandard life-style and a poor quality environment that constantly upset the homeostasis or balance of the body.

People are unwilling or fearful of changing their life-style and habits and would rather allow someone else to do it for them. Either the government or the physician is placed in the role of the father figure, who takes command when, in fact, the patient should take responsibility for his own health and the condition of his fellow man. This may be done through guidance, assistance, and example.

❦ THE BRAIN VS THE MIND

There is a tendency to equate the brain with the mind and certainly by inference the brain then controls the mind. This is most assuredly an incorrect interpretation. The brain is not the mind. According to the concepts of Robert Sampler, author of the book *The Metaphoric*, the brain is made up of two parts: the left hemisphere, which is the rational or thinking aspect; and the right hemisphere, which is the intuitive or creative side. At times whole societies traditionally function predominantly on one hemispheric wave length or the other. The people of the country of Israel, for example, as a whole tend to be more left-brain oriented—analytical, scientific—and have produced many scientists and new discoveries. In contrast, the Arabic countries tend to be more right-brained—emotional, intuitive—for their life flows according to feelings.

Your mechanistic logic is processed and acted upon by the left brain. You are able to reason within limitations and perform mechanical functions better. Consequently it would appear that the right hemisphere, being the intuitive brain, receives ideas from a spiritual force, whether it be that "wee small voice within" or an impression by a divine source.

It would seem that the majority of persons are primarily concerned with their five senses, which are constantly bombarding the left brain with nervous impressions, while the right hemisphere is mostly ignored. Within these circumstances the mind is ruled by the left hemisphere. Therefore, the physical world, with its limitations, is afforded the most attention and generally considered to be the basis for reality. Meanwhile impressions from the right hemisphere are frequently rejected because of the lack of appropriate reference for interpretation. We are dealing however with more abstract thought that lacks the limitations of the physical world and is infinite in character rather than finite or limited, as in the case of the left hemisphere.

I believe that seeking a balance of the two hemispheres is the ideal state. In meditation the left hemisphere is quieted to a degree that external nervous stimuli from the senses are filtered out. This allows impressions of the mind to be heard as an inner voice and at times seen in the form of symbolic pictures appearing in the mind's eye. Consequently, the real creative energy is released and exceptional ideas and concepts are received and subsequently impressed upon the brain. At this point the left hemisphere may analyze, systematize, and assist in a most important area, discernment of data. Discernment is the contemporary watch word.

The Bible reminds us frequently to go within for the kingdom of God. Meditation helps you to discern your inner self or God-self. Consequently you may expand your consciousness through this process.

An example from the past is the famous scientist, Thomas Edison, who was partially deaf and who made a habit of isolating himself in his laboratory for hours. He would emerge from these sessions with new ideas and inventions. Although he possessed a poor sense of hearing, he was a genius inventor, far ahead of his time, with over 1,000 patents in his name. In the late 1800s he developed the phonograph, the light bulb, and the electron tube, and perfected the motion picture projector as well as the stock ticker tape machine. It would appear that his loss of hearing was not a detriment, but an asset to this famous scientist.

Because he was a man possessing ideas far ahead of his time, I find his concepts in medicine very interesting and challenging. One statement he made is: "The doctor of the future will give no medicine, but will interest his patients in the care of the human frame, in diet, and in cause and prevention of disease." Nutritional therapy represents one way in which healing may occur and consciousness is raised.

❊ NUTRITIONAL THERAPY

One of the most remarkable studies to surface in the last few years was one by Dr. Ruth Harrell, professor emeritus of research psychology at Old Dominion University. Dr. Harrell conducted an eight-month, double-blind, placebo-controlled trial with mentally challenged children in Norfolk, Virginia, including a group with Down's Syndrome. She gave them a special supplement of vitamins and minerals and was able to raise their I.Q.'s 10.2 points over-all and as much as 25 points in one individual.

The daily nutritional supplementation used in Dr. Ruth Harrell's study of severely handicapped children included:

Vitamin A palmitate 15,000 IU
Vitamin D (cholecalciferol) 300 IU
Thiamin Mononitrate 300 mg
Niacinamide 750 mg
Calcium pantothenate 490 mg
Pyridoxine (hydrochloride) 350 mg
Cobalamin 1,000 mcg
Folic acid 400 mg
Riboflavin 200 mg
Vitamin C (ascorbic acid) 1,500 mg
Vitamin E (datocopheryl succinate) 600 IU
Magnesium (carbonate) 400 mg
Zinc (oxide) 30 mg
Manganese (gluconate) 3 mg
Copper (gluconate) 1.75 mg
Iron (ferrous fumarate) 7.5 mg
Calcium phosphate (CaHPO4) 37.5 mg
Iodide (KI) 0.15 mg

This study, one of the most outstanding, controlled, nutritional therapy studies in mentally challenged children, showed "a doubling of weight in treated children compared with those on placebos." There were also significant changes of the physical characteristics toward normalcy, including evidence of improved vision in three out of four children who wore glasses. The study, as published in the proceedings of the National Academy of Sciences, included a series of 16 children, ages 5 to 15 with initial I.Q.'s of 17-70. The physical changes noted were loss of the accumulated fluid in their faces, stabilization of cataract growth, which is quite common among children with Down's Syndrome, and improvement of muscular structure. Some children were transferred from special classes for the mentally challenged to regular public school classes as a result of the nutritional therapy. They had gone from hopeless to hopeful.

Of particular interest were the personality changes of the Down's children. Up to this time, children with severe mental disturbance were thought to be incurable. However when the therapy trial was complete, these children began to have a normal social existence. An example is one student who was told after completing eight months of his vitamin and mineral therapy that he used to be an idiot. He responded with, "No! What are you talking about?" He apparently had no memory of the prior years when his brain was not totally functional. It appears that with proper nutrition there is a potential for an awakening in some persons, a blending of the two hemispheres.

This possibly is where the term "half-wit" came from, for originally these children were only able to make use of one-half of their brains, their power to reason being severely limited to the simplest mechanical logic. However, the process in which the two hemispheres function harmoniously is a consciousness-raising event.

The late Dr. Roger Williams, professor emeritus of chemistry, University of Texas and director of the Clayton Foundation Biological Institute, put forth the genetotrophic hypothesis years ago. This theory supports the idea that one may have certain genetic deficiencies at birth that may result in mental handicap, as in Down's syndrome children. Interestingly enough, the ability to attain perfection, as is God's plan, may also be preserved in the life force of the individual. However, because of some structural problem, a human being may have difficulty reaching that perfected state. We may have damage in a biochemical-metabolic pathway that limits development, but once supported with a correct megavitamin, mineral, and herbal therapy, the pathway may be completed and the individual has an opportunity to realize his full potential.

For every disease that exists, God has given a cure — be it vitamin, mineral, herb, or food — that may be found somewhere on this earth. The individual must only possess an adequate life-force, a will to live, and the faith to seek the answers.

🌹 NUTRITION

Good nutrition is extremely important in achieving good heath. Certainly avoiding sugar must be considered one of the most important rules of nutrition. Even the Bible states, "It is not good to eat much honey." (Proverbs, ch. 25, v. 27) It has been found that too much sugar can upset the calcium-phosphorus blood ratio and thereby produce diseases of the gums, teeth, and bones. Also, the fluctuations in blood sugar, as seen in cases of ingestion of large amounts of refined sugars, may cause personality changes ranging from agitated, anxious, and hostile behavior to sleepiness and lethargy, not to mention fatigue. These symptoms are seen repeatedly in a condition known as "relative hypoglycemia." Even more interesting is the fact that other foods act on the body similarly to refined sugar. These foods are coffee, tea, soft drinks, chocolate, and alcohol. They may activate the adrenal glands that in turn stimulate the liver to release a stored substance called glycogen, which creates a rapid elevation of blood sugar. This is often followed by a significant drop in blood sugar.

It is important also to reduce the fat that predisposes us to arteriosclerosis. Dr. Ross Hume Hall from McMasters University claims that we should clean up our diet by avoiding refined sugars and starches and reducing our fat and salt intake as well as red meats. We must increase our intake of fresh fruits, nuts, and vegetables, and by simply doing these things we could eliminate most diseases within several generations. Consequently avoiding improper foods allows you to balance your body chemistry and therefore attain a homeostatic state, leading to good health.

🌹 RAISING OUR CONSCIOUSNESS

Many modern transpersonal counseling techniques, including biofeedback, guided imagery, and meditation, assist us in ridding ourselves of undesired habits. They also help us to better understand the situation in which we find ourselves and in directing the raising of our consciousness.

In the book, *Miracle To Believe In*, Barry Kaufman and his wife Suzi took a severely mentally challenged boy and brought him to a verbal and alert state. He was even able to master roller skating and bicycle riding. Using a therapeutic and educational technique called the Option Process, which requires the therapist's total acceptance of the individual to be treated, the Kaufmans spent a total of 7,000 hours in one-to-one therapy with the boy. The therapists totally enveloped themselves in his world, to the degree that they joined him in every bizarre behavior. Eventually by having an at-oneness with him, they were able to raise his level of functionality manyfold. His brain wave activity, as measured by an electro-encephalograph, revealed only weak and intermittent activity of the left hemisphere prior to the therapy and a relatively normal post-therapy function. An interesting unexpected effect was the improvement of the state of health and elimination of illnesses in the therapist; proving that as one heals intensely, without condition, one also becomes healed.

We have very complex regulating organs in our bodies. The hypothalamus is responsible for many regulatory mechanisms dealing with fear, anger, hunger, thirst, and temperature regulation. There are numerous neural as well as vascular connections between the pituitary gland and the hypothalamus situated in the brain. When a joyful and happy situation occurs, the hypothalamus sends messages to other glands, beginning with the pituitary. Consequently the appropriate hormones are released, leading to balanced body chemistry that then causes the appropriate action to occur. Therefore, when one is experiencing a state of joy, the appropriate amount of hormones are secreted and the correct biochemical reactions are completed. Good health is the ultimate result.

The classical example is given by the late Norman Cousins in his book, Anatomy of an Illness. He describes the frustrations of suffering from a painful, debilitating generalized arthritis. He was hospitalized and given the traditional drug therapy and suffered the typical stresses of being in the hospital. After several weeks he was told by his physician that the prognosis of his disease was hopeless. After much soul-searching, he checked himself out of the hospital and into a nearby hotel with a suitcase loaded with old comic movies, including Marx Brothers films. He also added vitamin C to his regimen. For three days he roared with laughter as he viewed these old movies and suddenly on the third day he became aware that for the first time in a long while he was completely free of pain and actually able to get a good night's sleep. Slowly he began to improve and started physical therapy, while always keeping a positive mental attitude toward his illness. He had decided to become more than a "passive observer." He became consciously active in his own health care. *The joy he experienced stimulated his body to act favorably and cure itself.*

While I was in Mexico in 1965, I studied at the famous National Institute of Tropical Diseases. There I witnessed an enlightening medical case. An Indian from a distant rural region was referred to the clinic. He was covered from head to toe with warts. It would have been impractical to burn off or otherwise remove the lesions as they were too extensive. After consultation among the staff, we made the decision to bring him into the room where most of the electronic and diagnostic equipment was housed and impress him with this labyrinth of modern medical progress. Being a simple man who was unaccustomed to these sophisticated surroundings, he was extremely impressed by the whole procedure. He sat in the middle of the room, attached harmlessly to the equipment, while several doctors turned switches and dials and caused lights to flash on and off repeatedly. This ceremony was performed every day for 12 days. At the beginning of each treatment, the patient was told that this was the most modern equipment available and that his skin would be cured. At the end of the treatments, sure enough his skin was 98 percent cleared; the lesions had simply fallen off. He was not educated enough to know that the wires weren't actually connected and weren't doing any physical good. But internally he was able to convince his physical body that this procedure would be a cure — and it was.

What we're seeing is the "placebo effect." Scientists are now finding that if a placebo, supposed to be an inert substance, is given and the patient is told that it will heal, in many cases it becomes an effective potion, curing the most complicated diseases.

The famous Dr. Albert Schweitzer once said, "Each patient carries his own doctor inside him," indicating recognition by this great man that we have a life-force operating in our consciousness.

Sometimes the patient must stand back and allow the healing process to occur. This isn't to suggest that the patient become a casual observer, but to consciously cooperate with the healing force and mentally direct the divine energy within to heal the body.

Consider the fact that a surgeon may make an incision to perform surgery and when it is completed, he sews the skin together. However, he cannot cause the edges of the skin to grow together; that process is directed by the divine healing force from within.

The human body is its own best doctor; it can balance itself and maintain homeostasis. It is the responsibility of the members of the medical profession to support this process and allow the body to heal. *There is no separation between mind, body, and spirit,* and I certainly feel these examples of the "placebo effect" prove this.

🦋 EXERCISE

Exercise has a distinct benefit in holistic health as well. Brisk exercise stimulates the cardiovascular circulation thus improving nutrition to the body and carrying off waste products. Similar benefits may be obtained from body massage if performed properly.

One hears the term "runner's high" quite frequently. Apparently, after running or working out for some time and while keeping the mind free of thoughts, the runner or exerciser is able in some cases to achieve an altered state of consciousness that is quite pleasant. One theory is that this may be the result of elevated levels of endorphins being released into the blood stream. These are endogenous chemicals secreted by the brain that block pain naturally as well as produce a feeling of well-being. Actually, what I have discussed are examples of holism applied to the individual, when body, mind, and spirit are united.

🦋 HOLISM

One may take the principles of holism and apply and expand these to the world as a whole. When a large portion of the world's population is malnourished and wanting, then an imbalanced situation is created and we have a world that is out-of-ease or "dis-eased." The world may be compared to the human. When an individual has a disturbance in blood flow, then an imbalance or disease is the result. If humanity as a whole does not receive their adequate share of food, clothing, and energy, then social breakdown is the product, and we have situations, such as conflict and rebellion, war and destruction of the planet, that can be compared to sickness in the individual.

Most people are involved in a struggle, day after day, simply trying to meet their obligations for basic needs: food, housing, and clothing and to pay their taxes and deal with the emotional needs of the family. Then, when they catch a glimpse of "light" or spiritual truth, they may become fearful or even repulsed. They have become accustomed to living in the darkness for so long that they have difficulty dealing with the "light." Not only does one need to recognize this as such, but it requires, in most cases, changing one's point of reference and life-style.

The planet earth is a great university of learning. We are here, experiencing many situations and receiving instant feedback that may be in the form of suffering. These situations may be stressful and painful but each one, no matter how difficult, offers great opportunity. If we deal with these circumstances adequately we may turn them into nonstressful, learning situations and realize personal growth as a result. Sometimes it is through illness that the most growth takes place. Thus it may be said: *There are no such things as problems, but only opportunities.* It is obvious, however, that at times it is difficult to change a challenging situation into one of enlightenment or learning.

❧ THE REASON FOR DISEASE

I believe I have discovered the reason for disease. At times we will have an accident, disease, or pain *inflicted* upon us. A time of incapacity or disability often ensues, necessitating rest. This enables us to take the opportunity to *reflect*—reflect on what we are doing improperly in our life path. Any deviation from this path is not in our best interest. If we take the time to reflect, we might become inspired. I believe *inspiration* comes from a higher divine source. We could discover what we can change or do to correct the improper patterns. If we don't do this, the illness may become worse, prolonged, or we may have other illnesses. The lessons get harder. If we take the correct *action, health* usually manifests. The mark of a good doctor is that he is able to help the patient reflect. Hence we must consider this process as an opportunity—an opportunity to grow and learn.

The following diagram describes this process:

DISEASE – HEALING PROCESS
Infliction $\longrightarrow$ Reflection $\longrightarrow$ Inspiration $\longrightarrow$ Action $\longrightarrow$ Health

God has given each of us freedom; freedom of choice, in all matters, even to give us the option of asking for His help or not, because God respects your freedom of choice.
—Annie Kirkwood

✤ THE CHALLENGE OF FAMILY

Another one of the most intense learning experiences we will have is in dealing with our own family members. This can be very frustrating at times, as well as very fulfilling. And yet, when in a recent Lou Harris survey Americans were asked what is most important in their lives, 96 percent responded with "Having a good family life."

✤ REACTING TO DIS-EASE

We are generally encouraged to avoid being in the now. Radio, television, and magazines tell us about pills to reduce or eliminate pain and consequently, ignore what our true selves are telling us. We suppress rather than adequately deal with situations. We fail to recognize what is really important or what really counts in our daily lives.

As I have stated earlier, the brain is more than the mind. Man is mind, and the mind is a creator. It creates the world that man or woman directs it to create. We choose our own realities. The society we live in has consensually agreed upon a collection of theories that, in toto, form an explanation of reality. This is called paradigm.

In the last 100 years the advancement of scientific thought has distinctly shaped our world through a linear thought process. We have evolved into a super technical society using sophisticated machinery, such as computer-scanners for medical diagnosis. Meanwhile the world continues to have greater and more complex problems, such as famine, overpopulation, severe economic and environmental disturbances and destruction. Then certain free-thinking individuals emerge from the population. These people believe that there must be new solutions to these enormous societal problems. If these individuals possess a balanced creative mind, they will perceive new solutions.

These courageous individuals put their toes in the water and test one new idea after another. Some are discarded, but some creative ideas are introduced and applied. Of course these pioneers may be laughed at, scorned, and rejected because usually the first one to introduce an innovative idea appears wrong. However, if he or she persists and ultimately more people discover the same or similar ideas, then these concepts are promoted more extensively. Today, using radio, television, books, and seminars, these new ideas may be rapidly dispersed. Next, research is conducted on the new concepts and positive data accumulates. More and more persons may know of the concept experientially as well.

Finally the data is so extensive and overwhelming that the majority of the population believes these new ideas and concepts to be valid. We then have a paradigm shift. Such is becoming true of our state of the world and the new holistic health and medical movement.

Several years ago, the prestigious American Council of Life Insurance of Washington, D.C., published a trend analysis program predicting the possible status of health in the future. The commission reported that "By the end of the 20th century most people will believe that physical disease was a symptom of some underlying emotional, mental, socio-psychological, and spiritual pathology." The report also stated that "there were few limits to an individual's responsibilities for his own health," and stressed motivating behavioral programs that "tap heretofore undeveloped powers of the brain and mind leading to a more vibrant life."

In order to live and grow we must have vision, dreams, and goals; otherwise, nothing is here to anchor our physical bodies. People need purpose in their lives and they are, indeed, looking for it. The holistic health approach utilizes education in an attempt to inspire, motivate, and assist in solving one's problems.

In conclusion, we should strive for three health goals: to be free of disease, to function at a high level, and, most important, to understand our true nature.

We may all become pioneers in this new movement. The time to take personal responsibility and to act is NOW.

REFERENCES

The American Council of Life Insurance. "Trend Analysis Program and Health Care of the Future." Report: Spring, 1980.

Anderson, Dr. Albert S. "Creation Metabology in Medical Practice." From *Natural Food and Farming – Official Journal of Natural Food Associates*, Vol. 27, No. 9, Atlanta, TX, March 1981.

"Closeness, Using Talent Rate High." From *The Leading Edge Bulletin*, Vol. 1, No. 13, Los Angeles, CA., April 27, 1981.

Cousins, Norman. *Anatomy of an Illness*. New York: Bantam Books, 1981.

Ferguson, Marilyn. *The Aquarian Conspiracy*. Los Angeles: J.B. Tarcher, 1980.

"The Foundation of Higher Spiritual Learning." From *The Inner Light, Holy Aeolus*, Vol. 1, No. 6, Wash. DC, April 26, 1981.

Friedmann, Terry S., M.D., H.P. "The Holistic Approach to Better Health and Higher Consciousness." Presented at the Second World Congress of Science & Religion, St. Petersburg Beach, FL, 1981.

_____. "The Holistic Physician." From *The Alantean Era*, Vol. 2, No. 23, P. 14, March 7, 1981.

_____. "Holistic Health and the Whole Man." Presented at the First International Congress of Parapsychology, Parapsychologie, Pyschotronque et Theologies en Comparison, Rome, Italy, July 1979.

Hall, Dr. Ross Hume. *Food for Naught*. New York: Random House, 1974.

Harrell, Ruth, M.D., and Ruth Capp, M.D. Paper published in the Proceedings of the National Academy of Sciences, Vol. 78: Jan. 1981.

"Hopeless Autistic Child Makes Startling Recovery." from *Brain/Mind Bulletin*, Vol. 6, No. 8, Los Angeles, CA: April 20, 1981.

Horwitz, Nathan, M.D. "Vitamins, Minerals Boost I.Q. in Retarded." From *Medical Tribune*, Vol. 22, No. 3: Jan. 21, 1981.

_____. "Retardation May Pose Genetic Nutrient Need." From *Medical Tribune*, Vol. 22, No. 5: February 21, 1981.

Kaufman, Barry. *A Miracle to Believe In: They Loved a Child Back to Life.* New York: Doubleday, 1981.

Kirkwood, Annie. *Mary's Message to the World.* Grass Valley, CA: Blue Dolphin Press, 1991.

Page, Melvin E., D.D.S. "Degeneration-Regeneration." From *Nutritional Development,* St. Petersburg Beach, FL: 1977.

Remen, Naomi, M.D. *The Human Patient.* New York: Anchor Press, 1980.

Sampler, Robert. *The Metamorphic Mind.* New York: A & W, 1976.

United States Senate. "Nutrition and Mental Health." Hearing before the Select Committee on Nutrition and Human Needs of the United States Senate, 95th Congress, Washington D.C.: June 22, 1977.

Williams, Dr. Roger J. *Biochemical Individuality: The Basis for the Genetotrophic Concept.* New York: John Wiley, 1956. Reprinted by University of Texas Press at Austin.

_____. *Nutrition Against Disease.* New York: Bantam Books, 1973.

CHAPTER 22

Reversing the Aging Process

IN 1994 there were 33 million people over 65 year old in the United States and this figure is increasing every year. In addition, the 76 million "baby boomers" are now reaching the age of 50. The trend in the United States is toward an older age.

Most doctors teach us that aging is inevitable. However, different cultures experience health and longevity beyond what is normally observed in our society here in the U.S. The quest for immortality has motivated explorers and dreamers for as long as we have recorded history.

The Greeks and Romans sought to obey the gods, who they felt would teach them of eternal youth. In the Middle Ages the Europeans searched for ambrosia, the food for the Gods that delivered eternal life. Spanish explorer Ponce De Leon discovered Florida while searching for the mythical Fountain of Youth.

What is happening today outside the United States? People in other cultures around the world are not only living longer then U.S. citizens but are productive in their old age. These long-life societies include the Vilcabambas, who live in the Andes mountains in Ecuador, as well as the Bilcabambas from Peru, the Abkhasians from Russia, and the Hunzas from the Himalayas.

To discover why a relatively large number of persons in these societies live to be 90 or 100 years, scientists have studied their life-styles. One of these researchers is Dr. David Davies, of the gerontologic unit at the College University of London. He found, first of all, that most of these infra-populations reside in mountainous areas above 5,000 feet altitude. Secondly, their lives are pretty simple and consequently stress free. Many do not have electricity and, therefore, no lights other than candles or lanterns. Their days are pretty much directed by the sunlight or lack of it. They get up in the morning and go to bed at night according to nature's light.

Next, their life-styles show that diet is unquestionably one of the biggest factors to longevity. Most of the societies with long life spans are vegetarian or they may eat meat once or twice a week. They also consume a low calorie diet.

Another factor is that they primarily drink natural spring water. This water is usually pure, free from chemical pollutants and other toxins. The spring water is normally rich in minerals and other nutrients. The next factor is exercise. Many of these societies lack convenient transportation, therefore, they walk. Many have their own gardens since food is not readily available, and they labor to grow the food.

The last factor that Dr. Davies found is their attitude. "Among all these communities with centenarians, there is a marked lack of interest in the area of death in general. It is as if death was a disease that never happens to them," he states.

If this data is valid and has significance as the cause of longevity, then societies who have opposite life-styles should have the shortest life spans. This appears to be true. The Eskimoes, Laplanders, Greenlanders, and Russian Kurds all have a life expectancy of approximately 30 years. They live in cold climates near sea level and they are essentially meat and fat eaters. Most of these societies have mechanized vehicles. Even the Eskimos now have snowmobiles.

THE AGING PROCESS

What actually occurs in the body as the aging clock moves ahead? Metabolism slows down, and the immune system becomes less effective. The digestive system is less efficient, and there is a decline in total bone mass. In general, the body's ratio of muscle mass to fat mass is 4:1 during youth, and 1:1 after age 70. The result is diminishing strength. Also, mobility and ease of flexion of the joints decreases. Memory fails more frequently, as does the ability to concentrate. The skin becomes thinner and, hence, wrinkles appear. Some people experience difficulty sleeping. Vision acutely declines, as does the libido.

Doctors currently agree that aging is the result of environmental influences and the effect of personal health habits on the body. However, doctors also recognize that genetics and hereditary codes determine our fate and influence our longevity to a degree.

Our genetic makeup is determined by chromosomes, which have coding in them called DNA. On the end of DNA strands are segments called telomere. Telomere act as a gene clock. In simple terms, the DNA acts as a template giving instruction as to how the body is to create new cells or repair damaged cells. Damaged DNA may give inaccurate information as to building new cells and hence one ends up with a dysfunctional cell. With the aging process damage occurs to the DNA. This damage may be caused by several factors, including the kind and amount of toxins in the body and the number of free radicals present. When too many of the DNA particles have been damaged and the telomere along with them, the cell ages and eventually dies. So this phenomenon is determined by the resistance of the telomere as well as the amount of damage occurring.

One feature of a cell is that while it lives it has metabolic functions. Oxygen and nutrients are taken into the cell and utilized and carbon dioxide and the end products of metabolism are discharged. These become wastes at a cellular level just as the body eliminates waste from the bowels, bladder, skin, and lungs.

Here are factors that determine the health or damage of a cell:

1. The amount of damaging products that come into contact with the cell.

2. The ease with which the wastes are removed from the cell.

3. The availability of the proper nutrients that may repair the cell.

So, by focusing on these three factors, can we slow down the aging process, or even actually reverse it?

We are living in an age of rapid expansion of knowledge. In the case of health and medicine, our understanding of the human body is doubling every 3.5 years, as I have said before. Today there is new information emerging that will assist us in turning back the aging clock.

I have created a two-fold approach to reversing the aging process:

1. What we can take into our bodies.
2. What we must do for ourselves.

Let's first look at what can we take into our bodies:

1. Drink Lots of Pure Water.

Americans in general do not consume enough pure water. With the abundance of other sugar drinks and caffeinated products, such as soft drinks, coffee, and tea, we choose not to drink water. Yet water is extremely essential for health. Seventy percent of the body weight is water. Blood is 90 percent water by volume. One of the benefits of water is that it carries nutrients and oxygen as well as toxins and waste products. Good water contains many minerals. So to have adequate nutrition or detoxify the body, water is essential.

Yet in our culture, water is a precious commodity. It is essential for manufacturing and agriculture, but the runoffs from these functions are polluted with chemicals, heavy metals, microbes, and other toxins. The healthy alternative for the body is ionized and purified water.

Most filtration systems merely remove chlorine and other impurities. Ionized water runs through an electrolysis chamber, which adds electrons to the water.

We know from medical studies that aging is caused in part by free radical damage to healthy cells. During this process electrons are removed from cells. In the case of ionized water it contains large amounts of electrons. This reservoir can be given to the cells so they become stable, hence reducing free radical damage and reversing the aging process.

Electrolysis also reduces the size of water clusters, from 10 to 12 molecules per cluster, which is standard, to 5 or 6 molecules per cluster. These smaller water clusters are much more easily absorbed by the body and are also easily transported. The net effect is better hydration of the tissue leading to less wrinkled skin and other health attributes related to better hydration.

Ionized water has long been used in Japan in private homes and hospitals. Now, as we become aware of the benefits of pure water, ionizers are being introduced in the United States.

In some filtration systems the water is changed to alkaline rather than acid, which is characteristic of most tap water because it contains many organic contaminants. One important function of a good water processing and purification system is to filter out impurities such as chemical toxins and microbes. Some protozoa can find their way through filter holes of three micron size. An example would be Cryptosporidium parvum. For this reason, in a good filter the pores should be one micro or less.

However, filtering does not remove all of the infectious microbes. Therefore an ultraviolet light system may be integrated in a water purification system. Ultraviolet light is a safe and efficient antiseptic system. It is one of the methods recognized by world health authorities to kill bacteria and other microbes.

Adults should drink a minimum of 6 8-oz glasses of water daily, more if you are detoxifying or it is hot outside.

2. Eat a Proper Diet.

What is a proper diet? We've all been told that we need a proper balance of carbohydrates, fats and proteins. However, the dietary needs vary depending on the individual, their weight and size, their metabolism and level of health. According to researchers, malnutrition is a major cause of death in nursing homes. As we age, the amount and efficiency of our digestive juices decreases. Also, foods in nursing homes tend to be over-refined and processed, certainly not organic. Hence, the elderly fail to receive as much nutrients from their food as younger persons do.

Here are some very important dietary rules, appropriate throughout life:

Reduce or eliminate red meat consumption. Toxins are fed to the animals by meat producers to reduce infection and to increase the rate of growth. Mass production slaughter houses increase the contamination of the meat and the amount of microbes. The high amount of toxins in animal flesh could increase the body's toxin levels as well. Recently there have been numerous cases of massive contamination by the bacteria *E. Coli* in slaughter houses. Even the meat that has passed inspection and reached our dinner tables contains an estimated 300 million bacteria per serving. This is in contrast to vegetables and fruits, which have an estimated 40,000 per serving. These products stress not only our immune system, but our hormonal system as well. This is a major reason we should strive to eat more vegetables and fruits or even become a vegetarian.

There is much scientific data that a high carbohydrate diet may shorten our life span. In th laboratory as well as in human studies, people who consume a high carbohydrate diet as compared to a balanced diet of protein and fats die at earlier ages.

Also reflected in scientific theory is that one of the causes of the disease process, including chronic degenerative diseases, and the aging process is the accumulation of acids in the body. Acid coagulates blood and could cause clotting. Acid accumulates in joints causing pain and arthritis. Acid contributes to the production of fats that accumulate with age. Chronic high acid levels eventually destroys or alter the cells. These altered cells can become malignant. Most acid conditions are produced by foods. Some of the acid producing foods are beef, pork, chicken, tuna, butter, cheese, peanuts, egg yolks, and oatmeal. Food that help keep the body more alkaline are beans, soybeans, bananas, carrots, potatoes, cabbage, egg whites, oranges, apples, and milk. So, if we can reduce the acid, we may improve cellular health and longevity.

3. *Take Nutrient Supplementation, Including Antioxidants.*

Almost everyone realizes that today foods no longer contain the nutrients they once did. This is because our soils, which grow the foods, are overused and deplete of nutrients. Of importance is that many Americans consume foods that are over processed. You may still hear an occasional dietitian claim that if you eat a well-balanced diet, "you don't need vitamins and minerals." Ignore them. This statement is not realistic.

So what nutrient supplement do we need? I will break it down into two areas: nutrients needed for detoxifying and cleansing; and nutrients needed for growth and for rebuilding tissues.

Detoxifying products include antioxidants such as vitamins A, C, E and the mineral selenium and the compound pycnogenol. Nutrients needed for growth, repair and sustaining the body are co-enzyme Q10, which strengthens muscles, vitamin B, and MSM. MSM builds protein from amino acids, helps growth of hair and nails, promotes healing, and improves libido and the elasticity of skin, joints, and tendons. It also retards wrinkling. Ginkgo biloba slows Alzheimer's disease and improves circulation, particularly in small vessels. A secondary effect of Gingko is better memory as nutrients are delivered more effectively to the brain. (I have used Ginkgo Biloba extensively in my practice to retard Alzheimer's disease and improve memory and circulation.) When taken after a stroke it helps the afflicted person to gain better function. Also I found that circulation of the extremities improved.

Carnitine, composed of L-Carnitine from tartrate, which burns fat and gives us more energy, and Acetyl-L-Carnitine, which optimizes brain function, are also important. Vitamin E, which acts as an antioxidant, also retards Alzheimer's disease. (M.Ernesto Sano, et.al., New England Journal of Medicine, 1997) Also, vitamin A and its precursor Beta Carotene (the class of carotenoids) not only act as antioxidants, but are builders and detoxifiers as well. "Numerous epidemiologic studies have demonstrated that individuals with the highest intakes of carotenoids—richly found in fruits and vegetables and/or high blood levels of specific carotenoids usually have the lowest risk for certain types of cancer." (*Veris*, Research Summary, Aug. 1997)

Glutathione is needed for detoxifying and cleansing the body. Its action is apparent in the liver, which is known as "the chief of detoxification." Everything absorbed and assimilated by our digestive systems initially filters through the liver. Long living and healthier aging adults have a greater level of glutathione in the liver. A recent study claims, "Low glutathione in the elderly may be a risk to problems associated with poor detoxification." (L. Lab. Clin. Med., 1992)

With aging, the ability to digest, assimilate and activate essential fatty acids is decreased. GLA (Gamma-linolenic acid) helps keep the skin smooth and has anti-inflammatory actions that prevent arthritis. DHA (Docosahexaenoic acid), another fat, is important to strengthen the eyes and improve brain function, and it may prevent degeneration of nerve cells. (Robert Crayhon, Total Health) Alpha-lipoic acid improves nerve health and contributes to the improvement of peripheral neuropathy and infirmity in which the nerves of the legs deteriorate and cause numbness and pain. This condition is often found in adult-onset diabetes. (N.E. Garrett, et. al., Letters, 1997)

Vitamin B_{12} (Cyanoeobalanin) levels were found to be lower in Alzheimer's patients than normal patients. (Johnston and Thomas, *Journal of the American Geriatric Society*, 1997) Also, it has long been recognized that one of vitamin B_{12}'s functions is to stimulate a good appetite, encouraging the aging person to consume adequate nutrients. Studies have also indicated that B_{12} improves the function of the nervous system and brain as well as the joints. Vitamin B_{12} deficiency is a very common problem within the aging population because of their lack of intrinsic factor secretion along with gastric juices. Intrinsic factor and gastric juices are necessary for the production and actions of vitamin B_{12}.

Essential minerals serve as building blocks and activating agents for other nutrients such as vitamins, enzymes, proteins, fats, and carbohydrates. One aspect of minerals is that they should be taken as a balance of the total number at a specific ratio. This diminishes the competitive absorption action that is common with minerals.

The mineral magnesium improves symptoms of dementia. It also strengthens the heart muscle and relaxes respiratory muscles, which may reduce bronchial tube spasm in asthmatics. Calcium builds bone. Iron builds blood and carries oxygen. Some reports claim that as many as 95 percent of the senior citizen population is deficient in zinc. Zinc deficiency may cause prostate problems, arthritis, depression, macular degeneration, poor appetite and taste perception, poor skin and nail growth and wound healing as well as a suppressed immune system. These are just a few examples of the macro minerals (those needed in larger amounts) needed for good health. There are also micro minerals, which are very important even though the total amounts are very small. Again, proper ratio and balance of both "macro" and "micro" minerals is important.

4. Increase Oxygen to Your Body.

We can live days without food or water, but only minutes without oxygen. Oxygen reacts with products of the body to keep it healthy and to continue adequate metabolism. This process is called oxidation, "the chemistry of life, " the process through which the body turns sugar into energy.

Part of the aging process is that the cells of the brain, etc., do not receive adequate oxygen. This is in part because of decreased circulation, which carries oxygen, or reduced permeability of the cell wall preventing entrance of the oxygen. Because of his research, Dr. Sheldon Saul Hendlen advocates breathing exercises and oxygen therapies to prevent diseases. The body uses oxidation as its first line of defense against bacteria, virus, yeast, and parasites. Adequate oxygen has been reported to help inhibit cancer growth. The cells of the body react to oxygen treatment by releasing important enzymes for cellular detoxification and for the utilization of oxygen. This process improves energy production and heals inflammations quickly by strengthening the immune defense system.

There are other ways to enhance oxygen in the body. Essential oils carry oxygen and deliver it to the cells. We may inhale the aroma of the oils, apply them to the skin so they are absorbed into the body, or consume them as an additive to our foods. (An example of the latter would be the essential oil lemon, which is added to food or water as a flavoring.) I recommend the daily use of aromatherapy and occasionally breathing exercises.

5. Take Enzymes.

Just as the life process depends on oxygen, it also depends on enzymes. While oxygen is fuel to the body, enzymes are the "go-betweens" that control the rate and speed of the energy output of each cell. They are catalysts. They energize you by helping to start your day and keep you going. They are needed for every chemical reaction in the body. Vitamins, minerals, and other nutrients cannot be used effectively without enzymes. The function of the immune system depends upon the presence of enzymes as well. Once microbes have invaded, the body works to produce the enzymes needed for the smooth operation of the immune system.

We have over 3, 000 different enzymes in our bodies. Some are derived from foods and others are produced in the body. The pancreas produces digestive enzymes, and the salivary glands produce other enzymes that help break down food so it may be properly assimilated. On the other hand, over 200 ailments are the result of lack of enzymes. For example, people who have cystic fibrosis lack the enzymes trypsin and lipase.

As we age, enzymes diminish. Tests have shown that 70-year-old people have about half the enzymes of 20-year-olds. Russian Dr. A. E. Leskavar reported, however, in an article by Dr. Marcus Welner, that "supplementation with enzymes increases the macrophages (cells that destroy microbes and cancer cells) by 700 percent and kills cells by 1300 percent in a short time." Some of the most commonly available enzymes are Papain, Bromelain, Trypsin, Pancreatin, and Amylase.

6. Keep Your Hormone Levels Adequate.

Hormones are products manufactured by the body that stimulate, regulate, moderate, and suppress growth and maintain the body's homeostasis. They determine gender, and they help us deal with stress. They also help to produce our physical structure, size, and shape. The major hormones that the body produces are:

1. Human Growth (HGH)
2. Dehydroepiandrosterone (DHEA)
3. Melatonin
4. Estrogen
5. Progesterone
6. Testosterone
7. Thyroxin
8. Adrenalin

With the exception of the last two, there is a major pattern involving the production of the hormones. Concerning the first six, the level of the body's production increases until the ages of 18 - 28, when they peak. After that, they decline, drastically reducing the body's blood levels. Some person's levels decline more quickly than others. I have observed 30-year-olds with low levels. Generally, though, the aging person has much lower levels then the 20-year-old. Could this be a dramatic factor in our aging process? It certainly has an effect.

The last two, thyroxin and adrenalin, generally maintain consistent levels unrelated to age.

Growth hormone plays a major role in the repair and upkeep of the adult body and, according to Dr. Elmer Cranton, "has such startling affects in older people that it alone may significantly extend longevity and vastly improve quality of life." It is essential for repair of tissue and organs. A cascade of events happen to a person who is low in human growth hormone. Muscle mass turns to fat and muscle strength decreases, bone density begins to deteriorate, the collagen of the skin breaks down making the skin thin and causing it to wrinkle, the efficiency of the brain function is reduced, and the joints breakdown and lead to aches and pains.

Taking HGH by injection will reverse these problems and keep one on similar performance levels as middle-aged persons expect. Furthermore it should extend life and make it more enjoyable. I have observed individuals in their seventies who appear 20 years younger and are exercising more and experiencing less fatigue. This happens approximately one year after initiating HGH therapy. One drawback is the expense of the injections, which average about $200.00 a month. However, I expect these costs to come down considerably as more persons learn of HGH and begin demanding it.

DHEA – The Wonder Drug

A newly published drug, DHEA, may be just the answer to a multi-use drug having little or no side effects. DHEA, the abbreviation for Dehydroepiandrosterone, is an adrenal gland hormone. DHEA is secreted by our own bodies.

It has been called the "mother hormone" because it is the raw material by which estrogen, testosterone, progesterone, and corticosterone are made. The DHEA level in the blood reaches its peak at 20 years-of-age and declines with age. Studies show that some people have premature low levels of DHEA. These people often experience loss of energy, declining function, and accelerated aging, as well as an increase in degenerative diseases. Conversely, studies show that having acceptable levels of DHEA can prevent or reverse many diseases.

Dr. Elizabeth Barrett-Connor, M.D., from the University of California School of Medicine in San Diego found a "48 percent reduction in cardiovascular disease and a 36 percent reduction in mortality from any cause" when the DHEA levels were increased to therapeutic levels. According to Dr. Barrett-Connor, the reason is that DHEA protects the body by inhibiting the enzyme Glucose-6 phosphate dehydrogenase, which normally accelerates the production of both damaging fatty acids and cholesterol.

Other studies reveal that significant diseases such as cancer, obesity, depression, high blood pressure, diabetes, arthritis, senility, and Alzheimer's can be either improved or reversed. There are also studies showing that DHEA may be significant in improving memory and stimulating the immune system. Yet other studies taken during weight-loss programs have indicated that DHEA may be significant in improving the fat-burning process, possibly by replacing fat with muscle tissue.

The best news is that studies reveal that if taken orally in prescribed doses, DHEA causes no toxicity. Because DHEA is an unpatentable drug, no pharmaceutical company is interested in informing us of its value and/or of marketing it. It is a not prescription drug, and a recent report from the FDA claims it may become a controlled substance. This means it must be used under the direction of a licensed M.D. and purchased from a registered pharmacist.

For this reason I recommend that a DHEA blood-level be evaluated prior to its administration to determine whether or not there is indeed a significant decline of the patient's DHEA level. A lack of DHEA could be the cause of the patient's illness, and making DHEA a dramatic and safe therapy available to the individual.

Melatonin is produced by the brain's pineal gland. It naturally assists in ensuring a good night's sleep. It may participate in controlling the aging process as well .

Evidence is significantly positive for continuing estrogen maintenance to keep the female body younger and also prevent heart attacks and other cardiovascular diseases. It prevents bone loss, combating osteoporosis, which leads to frequent bone fracture. It also prevents hot flashes and vaginal tissue thinning. Women should take natural estrogen whenever possible. The three estrogen derivatives are Estriol, Estradiol and Estrone. They should be taken together for best results. Today American women spend millions of dollars on these synthetic hormones.

PROGESTERONE — THE POWER HORMONE

Progesterone has many beneficial properties for the body. One of the major problems for women in our society is hormonal imbalance and its negative effects on the physical body as well as the emotions. We have seen an alarming rise in breast cancer in this country. This has been found to be related to increased estrogen levels and low progesterone levels as well as dangerous toxins and other chemical compounds in our environment. Also, fibrocystic disease and fibroid of the uterus are very common and are in part caused by these same hormonal factors.

A particularly disconcerting period in a woman's life is those years surrounding the menopausal stage. This may occur as many as eight years preceding actual cessation of menstrual periods. Not only could the menstrual periods be irregular, but the emotional problems may be numerous and include depression, lethargy, crying and weepiness, feelings of panic, frustration, irritability, anger, and mood swings. There may also be loss of libido. One of the greatest problems in western countries is the large number of patients who have hip fractures due to osteoporosis or lack of calcium in the bone. As a matter of fact, according to Dr. Jeffrey Bland, this problem accounts for the occupancy of more hospital beds than patients with other diseases.

Due to the large number of prescriptions of estrogen replacement therapy, it obviously doesn't help to prevent this problem and may in fact make it worse. The reason is that estrogen is a protagonist of progesterone. Also estrogen is given in high amounts, while progesterone is usually made in a synthetic state and is not processed well by the body. In fact, many scientists believe that progesterone rather than estrogen produces bone growth. Progesterone is also seen in

P.M.S. problems. Here, symptoms may include headaches, abdominal cramping, depression, irritability, mood swings, loss of libido, and water retention. Adding progesterone from the 16th to the 25th day of the menstrual cycle may reverse these symptoms. Progesterone may also reverse the aging process by accelerating the repair of damaged cells, and delivering more oxygen to cells, making them more viable.

One of the very important functions of progesterone is normalizing the immune system. It is particularly critical in this day and age when the body is being attacked by so many new viruses and so many antibiotic-resistant microbes such as bacteria and fungi.

Progesterone therapy is very effective in auto-immune diseases as well. In these cases, one reacts against one's own tissue. We see instances of this in some arthritis, systemic lupus erythromatosis cases, and occasionally in thyroid disease. Scientifically it has been shown that progesterone positively and significantly affects muscle tissue, blood vessel walls, the heart, the intestines, and the bladder. Yet many of the benefits of progesterone are only found in natural progesterone, according to Dr. John R. Lee. Synthetic progesterone, which is derived from pregnant mares and is so altered that it may not have the same effect on the human body as our own hormones, may cause detrimental side effects. Therefore, it is essential to use natural progesterone whenever possible.

In cases where the menstrual cycle and blood levels of progesterone are normal, progesterone therapy would not be indicated. When the menstrual cycle is intact, yet there are mild signs of progesterone deficiency, supplementation may be indicated.

Testosterone is the male hormone equivalent to the female estrogen and progesterone. Unfortunately, testosterone is practically the forgotten hormone. Unlike estrogen and progesterone, testosterone is rarely prescribed for men. Yet men complain of impotency with the aging process. By age 70, 20 percent are impotent. Prostate problems could be improved with proper doses along with natural products such as saw palmetto herb, which converts testosterone to its proper active form. Abnormal derivatives of testosterone cause enlargement of the prostate with aging. Much of the testosterone finds its way into the heart muscle, which tests show is strengthened by this great hormone. Just as the signs of aging—thin skin, energy loss, poor healing, muscle deterioration, and bone loss—can be reversed with female hormones, these symptoms can also be reversed with adequate levels of testosterone. Many physicians do not take the time and effort to test testosterone blood levels on their patients. If they did they would find a significant number with levels that are very low. Testosterone may be easily administered by injection, skin patches, and oral methods.

The last two important hormones listed, adrenaline and thyroxin, do not drop with aging as significantly as the others. However, both hormones need support. Due to many toxins in our society the thyroid gland, which produces thyroxin, is often dysfunctional. The consequence of this is premature aging, fatigue, dry skin, and lower body temperature, which translates into cold hands and feet. Replacement and support of the thyroid gland with thyroxin and the essential oil myrtle applied over the thyroid, assists in improving thyroid function.

With the amount of stress we are all subjected to, the adrenals take a tremendous beating. They begin to fatigue and are unable to keep up with demand. The symptoms of adrenal insufficiency are low blood pressure, fatigue, weight loss, and the body's inability to deal with stress. Again, supplementation may be indicated.

❦ How to Reverse the Aging Process

What are the things we must do for ourselves to reverse the aging process?

1. *Exercise Regularly.*
Statistics reveal that regular exercise is important for staying young. What is meant by regular? This is sustained exercising for at least 20 minutes at least three times per week. That represents a minimum. During the exercise period, if you are healthy, you should maintain a heart rate or pulse rate prescribed by your age and determined by the following formula: 220 minus one's age times .70 to .85 to determine the 70- 85 percent range of that particular maximum heart rate. Exercising three times a week is excellent, but if you extend the

frequency to five times per week, you may raise your HDL cholesterol, which is the protective cholesterol, and improve your fitness level. For men not only aerobic exercise, such as speed walking and exercising machines involving shoulder, abdominal, and leg movements, are good but resistant exercises work well. For women, in addition to the above, jogging has great benefits as well. With the question of competitive sports such as tennis, football, and basketball, etc., experts agree that in regards to age reversal, the jury is still out. Some medical experts claim it helps and others claim it doesn't. Some say it may actually be a detriment.

Along with physical exercising, stretching exercises are very beneficial. Yoga is another way to exercise and also to develop flexibility. It improves circulation as well as lymphatic drainage. You will receive better balance in your metabolism and hormonal secretion. It also stimulates the secretion of endorphins, which stimulates healing. This phenomena is called a "runners' high" because of the euphoric feeling that accompanies the action.

2. Maintain Proper Hygiene.
There are many things we must do to stay healthy. We should prevent infections from microbes found in contaminated food. Make sure the meat you eat is adequately cooked so that unwanted bacteria are killed. Water should be pure and free of microbes. Know the source of your water. Avoid drinking water from streams when you are in the wilderness. Many restaurants do not use filtered water, so bring along a bottle of the essential oil lemon. A few drops of lemon in your drinking water assists in purification and detoxification, and neutralizing chlorine as well as some microbes. At the same time, a few drops rubbed on your hands refreshes and helps clean your hands before you eat.

Public restrooms are a major source of germs. It should go without saying that you must always wash your hands after using the restroom. It would be prudent to open the door with a paper towel when you leave the facilities as door knobs are a source of infection. This is how infection is spread. The intestinal parasites and other microbes go from stool to hand to another person's hand to his mouth.

When eating at home, the following precautions are indicated: When preparing food, always wash your hands thoroughly after you have handled one food and are going to handle another. This particularly applies when handling raw meat. Also, always clean the kitchen surfaces thoroughly after preparing the foods. Otherwise, bacteria may be transmitted from one food to another. This is, again, critical with raw food. Food left over from a meal in your kitchen should be refrigerated immediately and not allowed to set and cool on your counter at room temperature. Use common sense; when in doubt, throw it out. These simple precautions may make all the difference of keeping you healthy.

3. Keep a Good Attitude.
Unless you deal with the traditional thought pattern that death is inevitable, the aging process is going to persist. As we witness death, this negative concept is reinforced. If you choose to die, do so in perfect health and vitality. Following this train of thought when we observe aging and degeneration occurring around us, particularly among our family and celebrities, it supports the concept of aging in our consciousness. On the other hand, growth and maturation is the healthy and acceptable process of our physical selves as we move through stages of life.

Until we remove the mental picture of aging and degeneration illness, we will never make substantial progress. We must not be so influenced by the negative thought pattern that is prevalent in mass consciousness. We must adapt a new paradigm that proclaims the degeneration and aging process invalid.

Our attitude is very important when dealing with anti-aging. If we have a positive attitude about our health and well being, we can overcome disease. When a person is determined to get well, the healing process communicated to the body by the brain and nervous system operates in the body.

Research shows that people with an attitude that challenges authority and demands exceptional care for illness survive longer then patients without this self-responsible attitude. People who are convinced they can heal and go to great lengths to support this, they have results.

4. *Cleanse and Detoxify on a Regular Basis with Saunas and Massages.*

A big part of staying young is removing toxins, such as heavy metals and chemicals as well as metabolites, which form as a metabolic end product, from the body. Many of these toxicities are deposited in the fatty tissue of the body. While this location lacks good circulation so the toxins are hard to remove, the location is at advantage when using sauna, both wet and dry. As the heat increases, the pores open up and perspiration intensifies, bringing the toxins out through the skin. One should take a 20-minutes sauna weekly for the best of health.

Massage is also very beneficial for many reasons. First, the masseuse milks the lymphatics, detoxifying the body. Second, thereby the tissues, muscles, and ligaments relax, accelerating circulation and healing. The therapist's personal touch sometimes allows for a sense of well being and further healing.

5. *Relax, Heal, and Regenerate with Meditation and Prayer.*

Studies show that meditation actually slows down the speed of aging and helps to regenerate the body. Twenty minutes, twice a day, is a wonderful way to assist in the integration of the body's functions and to assist in relaxation.

Certainly the influence of Dr. Deepak Chopra is significant. In his book, *Quantum Healing* (Bantam Books, 1989), he describes scientifically how meditation allows you to better control your bodily functions for improved health. In his studies, brain waves, blood pressure, and heart rate were measured in the laboratory. All were improved during and after meditation. The work of Dr. Dean Ornish is well accepted by medical authorities now. He has proved that yoga, a vegetarian diet, and meditation can produce a significant reduction in heart disease.

Prayer is a way we have to communicate with our Supreme Creator. As I and others have said, while meditation allows you to listen to God, in prayer you speak to Him. The writings of Dr. Larry Dossey should leave no doubt in anyone's mind as to the power of prayer. He proved again scientifically that patients who are prayed for repair more quickly from heart attacks, have less complications, and have a considerably lower rate of death than patients who are not intentionally prayed for. There should be no question about the benefits of prayer. Everyone should pray daily in their own way, regardless of their religious beliefs.

I would point out that the great contributions made in these areas were all made by medical doctors.

6. Use Affirmations and Visualization Regularly.

We should state daily those things we want to achieve. This is a method that helps make it a reality. When we hear ourselves stating something, particularly if there is repetition, our mind considers it a true fact. So if we wish the cells to regenerate and the body to remain young, we must state it. At the same time we are claiming these facts to be true, the body listens as a child would and obeys.

If we visualize ourselves behaving as a child would behave at the same time we are affirming this, it becomes much more powerful. Imagine yourself running through the meadows as you once did as a child. This works wonders in reversing the aging process. You may be able to feel it working.

If you follow these techniques, you will soon notice a difference in your being. We must continuously affirm, visualize, and assume that a long healthy life is a reality for us!

REFERENCES

"Low Blood Gr Luitathrone in Aging Adults." L.Lab.Clin. Med., 1992:120:720-5.

Chopra, Deepak, M.D. *Quantum Healing: Exploring the Frontiers of Mind/Body Medicine.* New York: Bantam, 1989.

Crayhon, Robert, M.S. "Slowing the Aging Process." From *Total Health.* Vol. 19, No.1: 32.

Garrett, N.E., M. Malcangio, M. Dewhurst, and D.R. Tomlinson. Neurosci, 1997. Letters 222:191-194.

Johnston, Carol S., Ph.D., R.D., and Julia A. Thomas, M.S., R.D., "Holotranscobalamin II Levels in Plasma Are Related to Dementia in Older

People," *Journal of the American Geriatric Society*, June, 1997: 45(6):779-780. (Address: Carol S. Johnston, Ph.D., R.D., Arizona State University, Tempe, AZ. 602-965-9011 (FAX) 602-965-6779

Sano, M., C. Ernesto, R.G. Thomas, M.R. Klauber, K. Schafer, M. Grundman, P. Woodbury, J. Growdon , C.W. Cotman , E. Pfeiffer, L.S. Schneider L.J. ThalJ. N Engl J Med. 1997: 336;1216;1222. A controlled trial of selegiline, alpha-tocopherol, or both as treatment for Alzheimer's disease. From *Veris*, Research Summary, Aug. 1997, pages 3-5, La Grange, IL.

Welner, Marcus. "European Scientists Say the Major Reason for Illness Is the Lack of Important Enzymes." Toronto, Canada: GeroVita Laboratories.

Appendix A

Cleansing

EMOTIONAL AND MENTAL CLEANSING

BECAUSE OF PAST emotional experiences, many of them traumatic and disturbing, we create blocks or patterns in our memory systems at various levels. When these traumatic patterns are removed, the our health improves dramatically. Here are modalities that are used for emotional and mental cleansing.

Aromatherapy
Certain odors stimulate recall of specific events that were emotional. Therefore, by triggering recall, one can get to the problem rapidly, identify it, and release it. (See Chapter 7.)

Hypnosis
In this modality, I guide the patient to relive the trauma. Remember, we record and at times suppress life events that are painful for us. We choose not to deal with them head on. By assisting a patient to experience the original cause of the difficulty he is able to get a better perspective on what really happened in the past. I assist the patient by dealing with the problem right there and then as if it is happening in the immediate present. This serves to clear the problem.

Visualization
Another technique to release emotional blocks is to visualize the problem, take a deep breath, and breath out while clearing the problem. Do that as many times as it takes to get the issue cleansed.

People Interaction

Another way to deal with emotional/mental blocks is to recognize them and realize that it is okay to let them go from your consciousness. This can be done by way of interaction and guidance from others. It could be a one-on-one experience where the therapist serves as a guide. Or, it could be in a group where a leader is present, but help is extended from all people involved in the session.

🌿 Physical Cleansing

We have years of accumulation of heavy metals, pesticides, and other chemicals and toxins in our bodies. Here are some modalities that help to clear away these toxins.

Fasting

In cases of severe toxicity a purging fast should be done to clean out the system. One such very effective fast consists of eating nothing but apples for three days. It is best to get organically grown apples. This dumps the poisons from the liver and other parts of the system.

Protein Purge

Another type of cleansing is ingesting a predigested powder drink to purge the system for you. The protein source of the drink is rice, which is a nonpolluting product that does not stress the body. The carbohydrates used are from Jerusalem artichokes, an easily digestible product that eliminates the need for the pancreas and other organs to operate.

Lymphatic Massage

Another form of cleansing and removing toxins from the body is lymphatic massage. The lymphatics absorb the poisons within the system. A painful spot on the body, whether muscle, ligament, or tendon, is quite often caused by toxic substances accumulated at that point. When a lymphatic massage is performed, it breaks up the unwanted substances and literally expresses or milks them through the lymphatic circulation system until they have been removed.

APPENDIX B

Recommended Reading List

SUGGESTED READING

THE FOLLOWING ARE BOOKS that I strongly recommend to anyone that has or is involved with someone that has any degenerative disease, is suffering from immune problems, or is suffering from stress.

Balch, James F., M.D., and Phyllis A. Balch, C.N.C. *Prescription for Nutritional Healing.* Garden City Park, NY: Avery Publishing Group, 1990.

Bieler, Henry G., M.D. *Food Is Your Best Medicine.* New York: Ballantine Books, 1982.

Brecher, Harold, and Arline Brecher. *Forty Something Forever: A Consumer's Guide to Chelation Therapy and other Heart-Savers.* Herndon, VA: Healthsavers Press.

Chopra, Deepak, M.D. *Ageless Body, Timeless Mind.* New York: Harmony Books, 1993.

Cousens, Gabriel, M.D. *Conscious Eating.* Santa Rosa, CA: Vision Books International, 1992.

Cranton, Elmer, M.D. *Resetting the Clock.* New York: M. Evans and Company, Inc., 1996.

Cranton, Elmer, M.D., and Arline Brecher. *Bypassing Bypass.* Herndon, VA: Medex Press, 1984.

Dyer, Wayne, W., M.D. *Your Sacred Self.* New York: Harper Collins, 1995.

Edwards, Ted L., Jr., M.D. *Power Aging.* 4201 Bee Caves Road, Suite B-112, Austin, TX 78746.

Enby, E., M.D., Peter Gosch, and Michael Sheehan. *Hidden Killers*. USA and Germany: Sheehan Communications, 1990.

Gittleman, Ann Louise. *Guess What Came to Dinner: Parasites and Your Health*. Garden City Park, NY: Avery Publishing Group, 1993.

Julian, James J., M.D. *Chelation Extends Life*. Hollywood, CA: Wellness Press, 1982.

Kubler-Ross, Elisabeth, M.D. *On Death and Dying*. New York: Macmillan Publishing, 1978.

McDonagh, E.W., D.O. *Chelation Can Cure*. Kansas City, MO: Platinum Pen Publishers, 1983.

Moyers, Bill. *Healing and the Mind*. New York: Doubleday, 1993.

Ornish, Dean, M.D. *Reversing Heart Disease*. New YorK: Random House, 1990.

Preston, Richard. *The Hot Zone*. New York: Random House, 1994.

Quinn, Dick, R.F. *Left for Dead*. Minneapolis: Quinn Publishing, 1992.

Redfield, James. *The Celestine Prophecy*. New York: Time Warner, 1993.

Robbins, John. *Diet for a New America*. Walpole, NH: Stillpoint Publishing, 1987.

Shealy, C. Norman, M.D. *Third Party Rape*. St. Paul: Galde Press, 1993.

Siegel, Bernie S., M.D. *Love, Medicine & Miracles*. New York: Harper & Row, 1986.

Siegel, Bernie, M.D. *Peace, Love, and Healing*. New York: Harper and Row, 1989.

Williams, Lindsey. *You Can Live*. Kasilof, AK: You Can Live Publications, 1996.

Williams, Roger J., MD. *Nutrition Against Disease: Environmental Prevention*. New York: Bantam Books, 1980.

Young, D. Gary, M.D. *Aromatherapy: The Essential Beginning*. Salt Lake City: Essential Press Publishing.

Appendix C

Glossary

THIS GLOSSARY IS INCLUDED to provide you with an understanding of some of the technical terms and words used throughout this book. The purpose of the book is to help you, the patient, understand the concepts and ideas being presented and not to turn you into a doctor, nurse, or other medical expert. Therefore, some of these definitions are in layman's terms rather than scientific or medical terms. This editorial latitude was taken wherever I felt that the "scientific" or "medical" definition did not provide a clear understanding. I don't believe that any of these inexact definitions will convey any serious misinformation.

Acetylcholine (ACh): An acetic acid of choline, normally found in many parts of the body, it is required for the transmission of nerve impulses.

Acetylcholinesterase (AChE): This enzyme, also called True Cholinesterase, is present in nerve tissue, muscle, and red cells and helps convert acetylcholine to choline and acetic acid.

Acidophilus, Lactobacillus Acidophilus: A "friendly" bacteria necessary for maintaining "bowel flora," digesting food, and preventing disorders such as candidiasis and thrush. It is also necessary for the production of certain vitamins, especially the B vitamins. (See **Bifidus.**)

Acquired Immune Deficiency Syndrome (AIDS): A disease that inactivates the immune system. This is a political and socio-economic disease as well as a medical problem. AIDS is a disease of the body, mind, spirit, and emotions.

Adenosine Phosphate: A natural substance that participates in hormonal activity.

Adrenal Gland: Gland located adjacent to the kidney that produces adrenaline and several steroid hormones, including cortisone and hydrocortisone that the body uses in stressful situations.

AHMA: American Holistic Medical Association, and Arizona Homeopathic Medical Association. Both AHMA's promote a philosophy that physicians in all areas of medicine can be holistically oriented. All physicians may benefit from a basic understanding of the principles of nutrition, exercise, and stress management, and should have a continued awareness of the physical, emotional, mental, and spiritual nature of the whole person while practicing in a variety of specialties.

AIDS: See **Acquired Immune Deficiency Syndrome.**

Allergen: A foreign substance capable of producing an allergic reaction.

Allergies: Adverse or excessive reactions to substances that do not affect other people. Recently, other terms such as "sensitivity," "hypersensitive," and "maladaptive reaction" have been used in place of "allergy." This is because certain foods and other allergens do not evoke the typical antigen antibody response that is commonly seen in allergies in which the body defends itself against foreign substances.

Allopathic Medicine: Modern medicine, the medical philosophy most prevalent in the U.S. today.

Alzheimer's Disease, Presenile Dementia: Mental deterioration of unknown cause. A new study indicates it may be related to accumulation of aluminum in the brain cells.

AMA: American Medical Association.

Amalgam: A silver-colored filling containing mercury in its composition. It is the most common material used in filling teeth today.

Amebiasis: This one-celled parasite may cause ulceration of the intestinal lining, along with bleeding.

Amino Acid: Chemical building blocks that help the body produce proteins.

Amyotrophic Lateral Sclerosis (ALS): A mixed upper and lower motor neuron deficit is found in the limbs. This disorder is sometimes associated with dementia, parkinsonism, and other neurologic diseases.

ANA: Antinuclear antibodies.

ANA Titers: A group of antinuclear antibodies used in the detection of systemic lupus erythematosus (SLE) and other forms of arthritis.

Angina, Angina Pectoris: A precursor to a heart attack. Symptoms include chest pain, arm pain, shortness of breath, excessive fatigue, leg pain while walking, discolored and cold feet and hands, weakness and numbness of the arms and legs, dizziness, light headedness, temporary loss of vision, and impaired memory.

Angiography: A evaluation method in which dye is injected in the arteries while X-rays are being taken.

Angioplasty: Opening the arteries by inserting a catheter and inflating a balloon while inside the artery.

Ankylosis: Stiffness or fixation of a joint by disease or surgery.

Ankylosing Spondylitis (AS): A type of arthritis where there is characteristically symmetric joint swelling with associated stiffness, warmth, tenderness, and pain.

Antibody: Technically, an immunoglobulin molecule that has a specific amino acid sequence by virtue of which it interacts only with the antigen that induced its synthesis.

Antibiotic: Kills or inhibits the growth of germs. Also destroys bacteria (good and bad).

Antigen: Substance foreign to the body such as plant pollens, fungal spores, insects, feathers, airborne gases and chemicals, food additives, preservatives and drugs, gasoline fumes, cosmetics, detergents, nylons, paints, insecticides, fertilizers, air smog or pollution, newspaper ink, common ink, felt-tip pens, and plastics.

Antihistamine: Drug whose function is to block the action of the histamine that does the damage in allergies.

Anti-Oxidants: Substances that stop cellular oxidation. Anti-oxidants are generally considered to be the vitamins A, C, E and the trace element selenium (ACES).

Arginine, L-Arginine: An amino acid. Its function is to stimulate the immune response by enhancing the production of "T" cells and protein.

Aromatherapy: The use of "essential oils" in healing and releasing emotional trauma.

Artery: A blood vessel that carries blood away from the heart to various parts of the body.

Ascaris Lumbricoides (Roundworm): A common parasite of the digestive and respiratory tracts that is said to be responsible for the deaths of 20,000 people each year.

Aspartame (NutraSweet): A synthetically produced chemical food sweetener.

Atherosclerosis: Plaque located in the lining of the artery wall. Commonly called "hardening of the arteries."

Axon: The material that process impulses away from the body of a nerve. (See also **Dendrite**.)

Bacteria: Microscopic germs. Some contribute to health; others cause disease.

Bentonite: A natural bulk laxative. Technically, it is a native colloidal hydrated aluminum silicate that swells to 12 times its volume when added to water.

Bifidus: A "friendly" bacteria necessary for maintaining "bowel flora" and the digestion of food. It is also necessary for the production of certain vitamins, especially B-complex and vitamin K. (See also **Acidophilus**.)

Blepharspasm: Uncontrolled blinking.

Bowel Flora, Intestinal Flora: The bacteria (plant life) normally residing in the intestines. (See also **Acidophilus** and **Bifidus**.)

Bypass Surgery, Coronary Artery Bypass Grafting (CABG): A surgical procedure (open-heart surgery) in which occluded (closed or partially closed) portions of major coronary arteries are bypassed with grafts from a patient's chest and/or leg veins.

Calcify, Calcification: To make inflexible by deposit of calcium salts (ankylosis).

Calcium EAP (Ethanolaminophosphoric acid): A calcium mineral linked to an amino acid, easily absorbed by nerve tissues. Appears to protect and repair the myelin sheaths damaged by Multiple Sclerosis (MS) disease.

Candida, Candida Albicans: A yeast-like fungus.

Candidiasis: An infection caused by an excess of Candida. Traveling through the blood stream, it can infect various parts of the body, ears, nose, throat, gastrointestinal tract, bowels, and vagina.

Carbohydrate: Compounds of carbon, hydrogen, and oxygen (CH2O), therefore the name. There are several types, though we are mainly concerned with the Simple and Complex and their different reactions in the body.

Carbohydrates - Complex: Starches, gums, and celluloses.

Carbohydrates - Simple: Refined sugar—detrimental to good health.

Carotid Arteries: The principal arteries in the neck supplying blood to the head and brain. There is both a left and a right side carotid and they each branch into an interior and exterior artery, providing a total of four carotid arteries.

CAT Scan: An X-ray image made by a Computerized Axial Tomography machine, where the areas before and behind the area of interest do not show, providing a very specific field of view.

Centrophenoxine, Lucidril: It reverses the aging process and removes abnormal fatty deposits (lipofuscins) from around nerve cells.

CFIDS: See **Chronic Fatigue and Immune Dysfunction Syndrome)**

Chelation: The process of surrounding or "capturing" a mineral atom by a larger protein molecule.

Chelation Therapy: Involves the intravenous injection of a compound called ethylene diamine tetraacetic acid (EDTA). This substance uses the chelation process to remove undesirable metals and minerals from the body. EDTA helps to prevent the production of oxygen free radicals.

Cholesterol: A chemical component of animal fats and oils called lipoproteins. There are "good" lipoproteins (High-Density Lipoproteins or HDL) and "bad" lipoproteins (Low-Density Lipoproteins or LDL). The ratio between HDL and LDL in the body is very important, particularly regarding the formation of atherosclerosis.

Choline: Acts as a building block of the chemical acetylcholine. One of the best sources of choline is phosphatidyl choline.

Chronic Fatigue and Immune Dysfunction Syndrome: A virus called "HHV-6 Virus" is thought to be responsible. Fatigue is the predominant complaint. However, this is not just ordinary tiredness, but exhaustion so overwhelming and of such long duration that it completely dominates and controls the victim's entire lifestyle.

Co-dependency: Two people dependent, one upon the other.

Coenzymes: A heat-stable molecule that must be loosely associated with an enzyme for the enzyme to perform its function.

Colchicine: One of the most powerful anti-inflammatory medications known.

Colitis, Colitis Enteritis: Inflammation of the colon.

Complementary Medicine: Using Holistic medicine to complement standard allopathic medicine.

Cortisone: A steroid hormone, manufactured by the body or synthetically.

CT Scan: See **CAT Scan.**

Cysteine, L-Cysteine: An amino acid with limited detoxification properties.

Dehydroepiandrosterone (DHEA): Produced by the adrenal glands, this is the most dominant steroid hormone in the body.

Detoxification: Removing toxins (poisons) from the body.

Dendrite: The treelike materials that process impulses toward the body of a nerve. (See also **Axon.**)

DHEA: See **Dehydroepiandrosterone.**

Diabetes, Diabetes Mellitus: A disease caused by an endocrine malfunction leading to high blood sugar. This is caused by two factors: an organ called the Pancreas that doesn't produce enough insulin; or that the insulin produced is ineffective.

Diuretic: Increases urine flow by forcing the kidneys to excrete more sodium, thereby forcing more water and urine to be excreted.

DMAE: A memory enhancing drug that also increases acetylcholine levels in the brain.

Doppler: Studies of the neck and extremities using sound waves.

Dysbiosis: Two organisms living together, causing harm to one or the other life forms.

Dysfunctional: Not functioning properly or at all.

Dyspepsia: Digestion impairment causing the feeling of indigestion.

EDTA: Ethylene diamine tetra-acetic acid. Used in chelation treatments.

Electro Auricular Acupuncture: Stimulating the acupuncture points in the ear electrically.

Electrocardiogram (EKG): A tracing made by an electrocardiograph.

Electrocardiograph (EKG): An instrument used for the recording of electrical voltages occurring during heartbeat. Used to evaluate heart abnormalities.

Electrolyte: Chemical substance with an available electron in its atomic structure that can transmit electrical impulses when dissolved in fluids.

Endocrine Glands: Miniature factories that produce hormones that regulate many body processes.

Endorphins: The body's natural painkillers are normally present in the brain and are activated by exercise, stress, mental exercise, and imaging.

Enzymes: A protein chemical that accelerates a chemical reaction in the body without being consumed in the process.

Epstein-Barr Virus (EBV): This highly contagious virus is a member of the herpes family and the cause of mononucleosis. The Center for Disease Control in Atlanta estimates that tens of thousands of people are infected. The symptoms resemble flu with fever, sore throat, swollen glands (lymph nodes), extreme fatigue, appetite loss, headache, aching muscles and joints.

Etiologic: Seeking to find or assign a cause.

Extracorporeal Photopheresis: Treatment using ultraviolet light.

Exudation: The escape of fluids from blood vessels and their deposit in tissues, usually resulting in inflammation or swelling.

FDA: The Food and Drug Administration, a department of the U.S. government.

Filariasis: A common parasite that causes elephant-shaped limbs and enlarged testicles.

Free Radicals: See Oxygen Free Radicals.

Flukes: A parasite found in raw fish that can be life threatening.

Gamma Globulin: Complex proteins that have sites of antibody activities involved in allergic reactions. (See also Immunoglobulin.)

Gastrointestinal Tract: Includes the mouth, esophagus, salivary glands, stomach, liver, pancreas, gallbladder, small intestine, large intestine, colon, and rectum.

Genetotrophic: Pertaining to genetics as it relates to body morphology or from hereditary.

Giardiasis: A parasite that resides in the bowels.

Ginkgo Biloba: An herb that stimulates the brain and improves memory.

Ginseng: An herb that stimulates the brain and improves memory, learning, and concentration.

Glucosamine, Glycosamine: An amino acid derivative of dextrose (sugar).

Glutamine: An amino acid found in the juices of many plants. An essential element in the nutrition of streptococci.

Glutathione: A tripeptide protein that is a powerful anti-oxidant, composed of glutamic acid, cysteine, and aminoacetic acid.

Gluten: The protein of wheat and other grains.

Glycothymolin: One of the most effective, as well as safest therapies for infections from yeast.

Gouty Arthritis, Gout: A form of arthritis characterized by excess uric acid in the blood. Uric acid crystals form in and around joints causing severe pain.

Heavy Metals: Includes aluminum, cadmium, gold, iron, lead, mercury, silver, and zinc.

Herb: A plant or plant part valued for its medicinal qualities.

Histamine: Chemical in the body that constricts the smooth muscles surrounding the bronchial tubes, dilates small vessels, allows leakage of fluids to form itching skin and hives, and increases secretion of acid in the stomach.

HHV-6 Virus: The virus thought to be responsible for Chronic Fatigue and Immune Dysfunction Syndrome. (See also **Chronic Fatigue and Immune Dysfunction Syndrome.**)

HLA-B27 Antigen: One of the hereditary "Human Leukocyte Antigens" genes that partially define the immune system.

Holistic Health: The AHMA considers Holistic Health to be a state of well-being in which an individual's body, mind, emotions, and spirit are in harmony with and guided by an awareness of society, nature, and the universe.

Holistic Medicine: According to the AHMA, Holistic Medicine is a system of medical care that emphasizes personal responsibility and fosters a cooperative relationship among all those involved, leading toward optimal attunement of body, mind, emotions, and spirit.

Holistic Medicine encompasses all safe modalities of diagnosis and treatment including the use of medication and surgery, emphasizing the necessity of looking at the whole person, including analysis of physical, nutritional, environmental, emotional, spiritual, and life-style values. Holistic medicine particularly focuses upon patient education and responsibility in the healing process.

Homeopathic, Homeopathy: The belief that healing must first come from within, accompanied by divine guidance. Like cures like; using a small amount of product causes a similar reaction as the disease to cure the disease. It is also believed that the body inherently knows what is good for it and if given adequate elements of herbs, vitamins, minerals, and all other nutrients, it will use them to maintain health.

Homeostasis: A state of equilibrium or balance of the body environment.

Hookworm: A parasite that causes anemia or deficiency in blood that may result in fatigue, poor appetite, and advanced shortness of breath.

Hormones: Chemical substances produced by the endocrine glands — thymus, pituitary, thyroid, parathyroid, adrenal, ovaries, testicles, and pancreas — that regulate many body functions.

Humoral System: Pertains to all of the liquids of the body, except blood.

Hydergine: used to increase blood supply to the brain, removing abnormal fatty deposits (lipofuscins), and promoting free radical scavenging. It improves memory, reasoning, and intelligence.

Hypertension: High blood pressure.

Hypothalamus: A portion of the brain that controls autonomic regulation.

Iatrogenic: Adverse conditions induced by the physician or treatment.

Immune, Immune Systems: Means "resistant to, or protected from disease, poisons and other agents." Our bodies tend to defend themselves against outside substances or particles foreign to them.

Immunoglobulin: A complex protein endowed with and functioning as a specific known antibody. It is responsible for the liquid aspects of immunity. It is found in serum, urine, spinal fluid, lymph nodes, spleen, etc.

Immunotherapy: A treatment in which a small amount of the allergy-producing agent is injected into the individual in increasing amounts over time. This eventually neutralizes the antigen, or attacking substance.

Interferon Beta-1B: A new drug that has some effect on slowing down the process of Multiple Sclerosis.

Intradermal: Injected just under the skin.

Intramuscular: Injected directly into a muscle.

Intravenous: Injected directly into a blood vessel or vein.

Kirlian Photography: An energy field associated with all living matter is photographed and measured. The force of the field is a reflection of the strength of the vital life force.

Krebs Cycle: A portion of the metabolic process where the carbon chains of sugars, fatty acids, and amino acids are metabolized to carbon dioxide, water, and high-energy phosphates.

Lactobacillus Acidophilus: See **Acidophilus.**

Lactobacillus Bifidus: See **Bifidus** and **Acidophilus.**

Latex Fixation Test: A laboratory blood test for rheumatoid and other forms of arthritis.

Leukocytes: The white cells in blood used for defense.

Lymphocytes: The white cells produced by the lymph glands. They are the cellular mediators of immunity.

Magnetic Resonance Imaging, MRI: A machine that uses magnetic forces to produce detailed diagnostic images of the body, similar to X-rays.

Malaria: A common parasite, responsible for killing more than one million persons per year and infecting 300 million others. It is transmitted by mosquitoes.

Mast Cell, Mastocyte: A connective tissue cell whose specific function is unknown. It contains histamine, heparin, and in some cases, serotonin. Mast cells cause much discomfort during allergic episodes.

Mediator: An arbitrator or go-between.

Minerals: Naturally occurring elements found in the earth that are inorganic (not animal or vegetable). Like vitamins, minerals function as coenzymes, enabling the body to perform its activities. They are required for formation of body fluids, blood and bone, and for the maintenance of healthy nerve functions. There are two types: bulk, including calcium, magnesium, sodium, potassium, and phosphorus; and trace, including zinc, iron, copper, manganese, chromium, selenium, and iodine.

Modality: 1. A condition under which symptoms develop. 2. The method of or the use of a therapeutic agent.

Mongoloidism: Down's syndrome; so called because of the facial characteristics of this condition and the similar genetic pattern.

Multiple Sclerosis (MS): A progressive, debilitating neurological disease. The characteristic pathology of MS is destruction of the myelin sheaths that insulate nerve, brain, and spinal cord fibers.

Myelin Sheath: A lipid (fatty substance) forming a sheath around certain nerve fibers.

Neurophyschology: A science that seeks to integrate the observations of the mind with the behavior of the body.

Neurotoxin: A substance poisonous or destructive to nerve tissue, especially an exotoxin that has a marked affinity for nerve tissue and causes degeneration of the myelin sheath.

NMR: See **Nuclear Magnetic Resonance.**

Non-Steroidal Anti-Inflammatory Drugs (NSAIDS): Used for arthritis and joint inflammation and pain, these include such drugs as Indocin, Motrin, Naprosyn, Feldene, Meclomen, Vicodin, and Clinoril.

Nuclear Magnetic Resonance (NMR or N.M.R.): This machine uses a massive magnet to measure the disturbance of the electromagnetic energy field that is found around all living things.

Nutrient: Essential substances that affect the nutritive or metabolic processes of the body, including proteins, minerals, carbohydrates, fat, and vitamins. They must be supplied by food since they cannot be manufactured by the body.

Nutritional Deficiency: the condition where one or more of the essential nutrients is missing or is not available in sufficient quantities.

Osteoarthritis: A type of arthritis marked by degeneration of the cartilage and bone of the joints.

Osteochondromatosis: A type of arthritis where a benign tumor consists of projecting adult bone capped by cartilage.

Osteoporosis: Brittle bones.

Orthomolecular Therapy: Restoring the optimum amounts of substances normally present in the body.

Oxygen Free Radicals: Unusually toxic oxygen molecules that damage cell membranes and fat molecules. They are highly reactive molecules with an unpaired free electron that will combine with any other molecule that accepts it.

PABA (Para-Aminobenzoic Acid): An anti-oxidant amino acid that is a base for folic acid. It acts as a coenzyme and assists in the use of pantothenic acid.

Pancreas: An large gland, located behind the stomach, that produces insulin and other digestive enzymes.

Paradigm: To show side by side.

Parasite: An organism living in or on another organism. It may be a symbiotic or cooperative relationship (both enriched) or a dysbiotic relationship (one or both worsened).

Parasitology: The study of parasites.

Parasitosis: The disease of having parasites.

Pathogen: A damaging organism.

Peptide: Any combination of two or more amino acids in which the amino group (having an extra electron) of one acid is united with the carboxyl group (carbon-based atom missing an electron) of another. They form the essential portions of proteins.

Phosphatidyl Choline: A good source of choline.

Pharyngitis: Painful inflammation of the pharynx (throat.)

Pineal Gland, Pineal Body: A small gland located within the brain that regulates certain endocrine functions and other glands. This important gland control such functions as blood pressure, body temperature, motor functions, growth, the reproductive system, sleep habits, and aging.

Piracetam: Is said to enhance learning and memory. It protects the brain against oxygen starvation, protects against memory loss from physical injury and chemical poisoning and promotes movement of information between the left and right hemispheres of the brain.

Pneumonitis: Inflammation of the lungs.

Polypeptide: Peptide yielding three or more amino acids.

Procaine, Novocaine: Primarily used as an anesthetic, procaine rapidly breaks down into P.A.B.A., a vitamin, and DMAE, a memory enhancing drug that also increases acetylcholine levels in the brain.

Protein: Any one of a group of complex organic compounds. Widely found in plants and animals, proteins are essentially combinations of amino acids.

Protein - Large Chain: Extremely complex protein compounds usually combining several amino acids and peptides.

Psychoneuroimmunology: The therapy whereby a person can activate the brain to stimulate the immune system to operate at a more efficient level.

Pulmonary Fibrosis: Progressive formation of fibrous tissue in the lungs resulting finally in death from lack of oxygen or heart failure.

Raindrop Therapy: *First:* Apply 3 drops of rosewood, tanactum and frankincense on each shoulder as well as 6 drops on each foot. *Second:* Apply 6 drops of Oregano and thyme in raindrop fashion from the base to the top of the spine. Lightly massage the oil into the spine using short, circular strokes about 3-4 inches long going up the spine. Oil once; repeat massage procedure 3 times. *Third:* Repeat with essential oils of basil, marjoram, birch, cypress and peppermint. *Note:* Drip the oils directly, applying only one oil at a time, with the exception of oregano and thyme. *Fourth:* Once you have applied and massaged each oil, then, with fingers slightly separated, lightly stroke upward and out from the spine, repeating three times. Repeat this procedure three times. *Fifth:* Massage cold-pressed almond oil over entire back, finishing with a hot compress. Apply a hot towel on the area in need using a plastic covered heating pad to keep the heat in. Use heating pad and dry towel with caution.

Regional Enteritis, Regional Ileitis, Crohn's Disease: A chronic inflammation of the bowel wall frequently leading to intestinal blockage.

Reiter's Syndrome: A disease of unknown cause, but not caused by gonorrhea, occurring predominately in males, causing inflammation of the urethra followed by inflammation of the eye or eyelid and arthritis.

Rheumatoid Arthritis, Rheumatism: A variety of disorders marked by inflammation or degeneration of the joints and related structures. It is accompanied by pain, stiffness, and/or limited motion of these parts.

Salmonella: A bacteria of which typhoid is one. More than a thousand types have been identified.

Schistosomiasis: An infection of schistosoma parasites that severely affects 20 million victims in Africa, Asia, and South America.

Serous Otitis Media: Presence of fluid in the middle ear, with or without infection.

Steroids: A group name for hormones generally produced by the adrenal glands that contain a hydrogenated cyclopentophenanthrene-ring system. These include cortisone, progesterone, adrenocortical hormones, bile acids, and sterols, such as cholesterol.

Sulfonylurea: A medication used in the treatment of mild cases of diabetes.

Symbiosis: Denotes two organisms living together with benefit to both life forms.

Systems of the Body: A series of interconnected parts that function together in a common purpose. Some of the major systems in the human body are:

Bowel Filtering: A system consisting of the lower portion of the digestive system and including the large intestines, small intestines, colon, and rectum.

Circulatory: The vessels conveying blood to the entire body.

Defense: A system that protects the body.

Digestive: The organs associated with the ingestion, digestion, and absorption of food.

Immune: A combination of cells, proteins, glands, and organs that fight foreign substances such as viruses and harmful bacteria.

This system includes the liver, spleen, thymus, bone marrow, and the lymphatic system.

Lymphatic: An important part of the immune system, it includes the lymph glands, lymph vessels, and clear fluid flowing throughout the body. It nourishes tissue and returns waste matter to the blood stream.

Nervous: Combining the central and peripheral nervous systems, it is composed of the brain, spinal cord, nerves, and ganglia (groups of nerves).

Respiratory: The group of organs by which gases are exchanged between the ambient air and the blood. These include the nose, mouth, epiglottis, trachea, bronchial tubes, lungs, and diaphragm.

Urogenital: Includes the organs concerned with the production and elimination of urine and the reproductive organs.

Systemic: Pertaining to or affecting the body as a whole.

Systemic Lupus Erythematosus, Lupus (SLE): A general connective tissue disorder affecting mainly middle-aged women and characterized by mild to severe skin eruptions.

Thrush: An yeast infection (candidiasis) of the mouth, generally in infants.

Thymus Gland: A gland vitally important in initiating immune response, to create antibodies to overcome disease, increase our interferon and improve our defense system, and combat diseases.

Toxic: Poison.

Toxicity: Poisonous reaction that impairs body functions and/or damages cells.

Trauma: A wound or injury, whether physical or psychic (emotional.)

Traumatic Arthritis: Arthritis caused by a trauma or injury.

Tryptophan: An amino acid existing in proteins, it is essential for growth of infants and maintaining nitrogen equilibrium in adult bodies. It has been used for sedation and sleep therapy.

Typhoid, Typhoid Fever: An acute infection caused by Salmonella bacteria. Often caused by contaminated water and may cause death in 4 to 14 days

Ulcerative Colitis: Chronic, reoccurring ulceration of the colon of unknown cause. It is characterized by cramping abdominal pain, rectal bleeding, and loose discharges of blood, pus, and mucus.

Ultrasound: A machine using low-frequency sound waves, producing diagnostic pictures similar to X-rays.

Vaginitis: Inflammation of the vagina, vaginal infection.

Vanadyl Sulfate: A mineral compound made from the metal Vanadium, that may lower blood sugars naturally.

Vein: A blood vessel that returns blood to the heart.

VIP: Vasoactive Intestinal Polypeptide - A chemical secreted by the intestine.

Vitamin: A general term for a number of unrelated organic substances that are necessary for the normal metabolic functioning of the body.

Vitamin B-5 (Pantothenic Acid): Helps convert choline to acetylcholine.

Wellness: A lack of illness with a feeling of well being.

Whipples' Disease: A malabsorption syndrome, where the body cannot absorb nutrients.

Yeast, Yeast Fungus: A single-cell organism that can cause infection of the skin, mouth, vagina, rectum, and other parts of the gastrointestinal system and body. (See also **Candida**.)

REFERENCES:

Balch, James F., MD, and Phyllis A. Balch, CNC. *Prescription for Nutritional Healing*. Garden City Park, NY: Avery Publishing Group, 1990

Dorland's Illustrated Medical Dictionary, Twenty-fifth Edition. Philadelphia: W.B. Saunders Company, 1975.

Griffith, H. Winter, MD. *Complete Guide to Vitamins, Minerals & Supplements*. Tucson, AZ: Fisher Books, 1988.

Henry, John Bernard, MD. *Clinical Diagnosis & Management by Laboratory Methods*. Philadelphia: W.B. Saunders Company, 1991.

Julian, James J., MD. *Chelation Extends Life*. Hollywood, CA: Wellness Press, 1982.

The Medical & Health Sciences Word Book, Second Edition. Boston: Houghton Mifflin, 1982.

Webster's Medical Speller. Springfield, MA: Merriam-Webster Inc., 1975.

Webster's Ninth New Collegiate Dictionary, Springfield, MA: Merriam-Webster Inc., 1984.

Appendix D

Commentaries

Dr. Terry Shepherd Friedmann, M.D.
My reward is seeing profound changes in my patients!

Charles Collins, Stroke Patient

It was May of 1992 and I was 53 years old when I had my first stroke. I was working at my home/office computer at the time. I suddenly felt very odd and then collapsed and fell off of my chair to the floor, unable to move. After about a half hour, I regained control of my left side and was able to crawl to the couch and lie down. After about two hours I regained control of my right side, although I was very, very weak.

An angiogram showed that I had a complete blockage of the left interior carotid artery. This is one of two major arteries supplying blood to the brain. The other (the right interior carotid artery) goes up the right side of the neck. According to the angiogram, it was the one supplying nearly all of the blood to my brain, which as owner of a computer consulting company, I need to use frequently.

For several months after this major stroke, I continued to have minor strokes, called TIAs, two to four times a day. They varied in severity, from a weakness in the right side (not being able to lift anything), to involuntary muscle spasms where my right arm and/or leg would twitch or move on their own. Initially, during these severe attacks, if I happened to be standing or walking, I would suddenly fall. Gradually I learned to anticipate an attack in time to sit down quickly. These attacks would last anywhere from 20 minutes to two hours each. Of course, this was completely incapacitating.

I met Dr. Friedmann the first week in September, after suffering with these daily attacks for nearly four months. He started me on EDTA chelation therapy immediately. At his insistence, I also completely changed my lifestyle. I instantly quit my smoking habit of three packs a day for over 35 years. To quit, I used a combination of "the patch," hypnotherapy supplied by Dr. Friedmann, and my desire to live. I needed to lose weight (30 pounds)and lower my cholesterol and triglycerides. With tremendous help from my wife, I changed my diet completely. I stopped eating all red meat, fried foods, and dairy products, and reduced my intake of sugar and salt drastically. I also started a daily regimen of vitamins, minerals, and herbs.

My last stroke of any magnitude whatsoever was on October 10, after 15 chelation treatments. Because of the danger involved, I have not had another cranial angiogram. I don't believe that the blockage in my left carotid artery is gone. However, I believe that the combination of the chelation, diet, vitamins, etc., has substantially increased the blood flow through the right side carotid and other arteries. This therapy appears to have completely eliminated the strokes and TIAs, since I have not had one in months.

Rose Ludwich, Diabetes Patient

Chelation therapy administered by Dr. Friedmann may very well have saved my job.

An air traffic controller, I was decertified monthly for diabetes. I was on maximum oral dosage of Diabeta, which never brought my blood sugar down to a level acceptable to the Federal Aviation Administration flight surgeon. I was told by management that I would probably have to go on insulin if I wanted to finish my career. This was unacceptable to me, and so, chelation therapy began.

After 11 treatments my medication was cut in half. After eight more, I was down to 5 mg. and following the next treatment, was off medication completely.

I was then recertified by the FAA and regained my job as an air traffic controller. I now submit a report of my blood sugar once every three months, with no fear of decertification. I am told that I will probably be extended to a six month recheck period. I don't think management believes it, but the medical record speaks for itself— and the figures don't lie!

INDEX